To Marina

Enjoy the book &
the journey

Steve Hodder
Oct 7 2010

Meta-Physician on Call for Better Health

Meta-Physician on Call for Better Health

Metaphysics and Medicine for Mind, Body and Spirit

Steven E. Hodes, M.D.

Practical and Applied Psychology
Judy Kuriansky, Series Editor

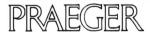

Westport, Connecticut
London

Library of Congress Cataloging-in-Publication Data

Hodes, Steven E., 1948–
    Meta-physician on call for better health : metaphysics and medicine for mind, body, and spirit /
Steven E. Hodes.
        p. ; cm.—(Practical and applied psychology, ISSN 1938–7725)
    Includes bibliographical references and index.
    ISBN-13: 978–0–313–34839–6 (alk. paper)
        1. Holistic medicine.   2. Mind and body.   3. Medicine, Psychosomatic.   4. Metaphysics.
[DNLM: 1. Holistic Health.   2. Metaphysics.   3. Mind-Body Relations (Metaphysics).
4. Psychosomatic Medicine—methods.   5. Spirituality. W 61 H687m 2008]   I. Title.   II. Series.
    R733.H613   2008
    613–dc22   2007031628

British Library Cataloguing in Publication Data is available.

Library of Congress Catalog Card Number: 2007031628
ISBN-13: 978–0–313–34839–6
ISSN: 1938–7725

First published in 2008

Praeger Publishers, 88 Post Road West, Westport, CT 06881
An imprint of Greenwood Publishing Group, Inc.
www.praeger.com

Printed in the United States of America

The paper used in this book complies with the
Permanent Paper Standard issued by the National
Information Standards Organization (Z39.48–1984).

10 9 8 7 6 5 4 3 2 1

To William James (1842–1910)
for his courage to pursue metaphysical truth
in the face of the critics of his day

META-PHYSICIAN'S MOTTO

Do not believe what you have heard.
Do not believe in tradition because it is handed down many generations.
Do not believe in anything that has been spoken of many times.
Do not believe because the written statements come from some old sage.
Do not believe in conjecture.
Do not believe in the authority of teachers or elders.
But after careful observation and analysis, when it agrees with reason and it will
    benefit one and all, then accept it and live by it.

—The Buddha, Gautama Siddhartha

Contents

Part V: Spiritual View on the Nature of Life: Inspirations from Kabbalah and Buddha

Part VI: Choosing Healing as a Way of Life

Part VII: Dr. Steve's Prescriptions for Calling Forth Your Inner Meta-Physician

Series Foreword

Everyone dreams of having a doctor with a heart. Dr. Steven Hodes is such a doctor. Here is a book that is as enjoyable as reading a novel for anyone who is—or has ever been—a patient (virtually all of us). But it is also a book for professionals, and aspiring professionals, who are willing to expand their traditional role to embrace a more spiritual approach to holistic healing.

The field of complementary and alternative medicine was introduced about two decades ago, championed by the noted surgeon Dr. Bernie Siegel. His book *Love, Medicine & Miracles* invited patients and physicians to explore dreams and imagery as part of a more enlightened way to live with illness, and to die in dignity. His ideas at that time were revolutionary but everyone fell in love with "Bernie" (as he likes to be called). Dr. Hodes picks up where Bernie left off. He takes us on a journey of his transformation as a Phi Beta Kappa graduate in religious studies who went on to get his M.D. degree at a highly respected medical school—Albert Einstein College of Medicine—to become a respected practitioner of gastrointestinal medicine (or, as it is called, a "GI man"). Over the years of his practice, Dr. Hodes gradually looked into his own soul to reflect on what healing is really about and discovered the importance of the connection between body, mind, and spirit. It's a tripartite connection that I, as a psychologist, believe is the key to health—and happiness.

Yet, Dr. Hodes does not try to force his view of a "meta-physician" on anyone. In fact, he continually advises us to be an open-minded skeptic about embracing a more spiritual approach to medicine that merges faith with fact. While I appreciate his empowering us to question, I am already convinced of the value of the integration of science with spirituality.

People of all ages today are increasingly concerned about not only maintaining a fit body but also emotional well-being. Consequently, they are more receptive to new ideas. Imagine a doctor willing to consider the impact on your illness of your past lives or your karma (the concept that your life today is affected by your past and influences your future), and willing to explore with you about your soul's destiny in life—and in death.

I appreciate Dr. Steve's combination of the rational and reasoned with the expanded and enlightened, being grounded in science but open to the spirit. I also enjoy his view of healing as a combination of gratitude, forgiveness, and accepting all emotions from happiness to sadness. And I am touched by his stories of people handling their pain, who prove the point that we control our health by what we think and believe. As a psychologist who has spent years working alongside doctors, I hope my colleagues will think more like Dr. Hodes. And as a person, I want my doctors to be capable and also compassionate, like Dr. Steve.

Dr. Judy Kuriansky
Series Editor, Practical and Applied Psychology

Acknowledgments

Many people were instrumental in the realization of this book. There were the many patients who openly shared their personal problems, allowing me to come to the understanding that their physical complaints were manifestations of an imbalance between mind, body, and spirit. Their deeply personal anecdotes of spiritual and paranormal encounters provided vivid evidence for me of a deep reality beyond the obvious. I honor their gift to me—the privilege of allowing me to participate in their healing process.

Likewise, I must acknowledge the many encounters with nurses, staff, friends, and acquaintances who offered me glimpses into their highly personal—and often confusing but deeply compelling—experiences. Most confided that they had shared these stories with few others out of fear of ridicule. This only encouraged me further to acknowledge their validity.

I must to express thanks to my students in Contemporary Metaphysics at Brookdale College in Lincroft, New Jersey. They challenged me to learn before I could call myself a "teacher" and have shared their own incredible experiences with me as well.

I am grateful to Rev. Laurie Sue Brockway, an experienced author and editor who has been my guide and advisor throughout this process. Her knowledge, compassion, and inspiration encouraged me to continue to seek my highest destiny. It was through her association with Dr. Judy Kurianksy, editor of the Practical and Applied Psychology Series for Praeger, that this book came to attention of Debbie Carvalko, who welcomed the book and did all she could to bring it to fruition. I am deeply indebted to them all.

I also acknowledge my family: my sister Carol, my children Jaclyn and Seth, and my parents. In the early stages of this book, both my parents became seriously ill. My father, Frank, came back from death's doorstep to be with my mother for her final days. My Mother Mildred died after a progressive illness. My Dad's miraculous recovery supplied me with a powerful motivation to attempt to make sense of this chaotic personal universe we all inhabit ... and to write about it with the intention to help others.

And finally, I express my appreciation for the love and support of my wife of thirty-five years and best friend Ardith. When we took our marriage vows "for better or worse," we had no idea that we would later have to add the line "And I promise to be patient and encouraging as you undertake the massive project of writing a book!"

Introduction

What is Metaphysics: "The philosophical investigation of the nature, constitution, and structure of reality."

Who is a Metaphysician: "a practitioner or student of (the above)."
—The Cambridge Dictionary of Philosophy

What is a Meta-Physician: a physician who has been changed or transformed (Greek prefix *meta*) by his own personal journey.
—S.E. Hodes, M.D.

This is a book about my personal metaphysical journey. Yet I truly believe you will find it meaningful as an approach to better health and well-being in your own life. Each chapter in this book represents a metaphysical theme that is part of my overall prescription for living.

As members of this strange and complex species, we are all seeking answers to the great questions of existence: Why are we here? Is there a purpose or meaning to life? Why do we live in fear and worry so much of the time? Can we create positive change in our lives, or are we like the wind-blown fallen leaves, living and dying by the whim of chance and circumstance? Is there any reason to be optimistic about what lies ahead for us?

As someone who has been dealing with the health of the physical body for over thirty years, I have turned my focus to that of the mind and spirit as well. I did so out of an innate curiosity about the way the universe works and in the process rediscovered what it meant to truly be a healer.

Not to anyone's surprise, it is all about the same thing—recognizing and creating our own reality through an awareness of what exists and what is. This is the meaning of metaphysics. It is not about bizarre and esoteric ideas. It is about how we live our lives, here and now.

The good news is this: we are all capable of uncovering the meta-physician within. Sometimes we need a bit of guidance from others who have begun their own journey and can show us the way. Ultimately it is not about following others, their path, their beliefs, or their practices. I would hope the material I share in this book simply shines a light on the path so you can begin to see where you are going as you take those first steps.

The journey is all about taking charge of your own destiny, your own health, by recognizing that

1. You are entitled to do so.
2. You are capable of learning how.
3. You are able to achieve the highest level of peace and healing possible.

METAPHYSICS IS AT THE CORE OF REALITY

Close to forty years ago I turned my back on religious studies to pursue the study of the physical body, within the domain of medicine. These many years later, I have rediscovered the metaphysical core of my being. It has led me back to the reality that true healing is the synthesis of mind, body, and spirit.

As a physician, I have spent the better part of nearly thirty years listening to the complaints of patients, making an assessment of their condition and offering prescriptions for treatment. As a meta-physician, I continue to utilize a systematic approach with people who need healing, but I do so with a broader base of resources. As a meta-physician, I explore more deeply the emotional and psychological states of being of patients. I can call upon their religious and spiritual beliefs as tools in helping me help them with their problems.

Metaphysics is an oft-used, yet often misunderstood, concept. It is frequently utilized as an umbrella term for "New Age" thinking, magic, the paranormal, the occult. In truth, by definition, it is the branch of philosophy that endeavors to study the nature of reality.

But as I see it, we do not have to be academic philosophers to embrace metaphysics. Not only are studies of the paranormal and spiritual aspects of metaphysics within this context, but so are science and art as well. In general, *any* effort to characterize and understand the way the universe works has metaphysical implications.

The prefix *meta* in *metaphysics* is derived from the Greek for *above* because Aristotle's writings on what he called his First Philosophy were discovered centuries later above his writings on the physical world. Therefore, we are ALL meta-physicians.

I have adopted another meaning of the Greek prefix *meta*. It also refers to change or transformation. Because my belief about life and healing has been transformed by my own journey, and because my transformation has impacted those I touch, I refer to myself as a meta-physician.

However, do not for a moment believe that metaphysics is a pursuit just for me, or for the full-time philosopher, dreamer, or mystic alone. Metaphysics, in fact, is *nothing less than* the basis for what we all believe to be real. And I can guarantee you, we all have very personal, individualized ways of looking at the world. The meta-physician, however, creates not only his or her own way of seeing things but his or her own reality. Our metaphysical perspective is the lens through which all that surrounds us is understood. There is no other way to define what is real.

A meta-physician is a person who knows it is ultimately about how we live our lives on a daily basis, and that it is absolutely crucial that we spend time assessing and reflecting on what we believe.

For many, religion offers the basis for their metaphysical beliefs. For many, it offers the "whole package"—what to believe; what is true; what moral values one should adopt; and which rituals, prayers, and traditions will assist in traversing life's passages. In some faiths, negative or disturbing events may be viewed as some kind of punishment for sin. On the other hand, for those who are essentially free of religious dogma, experiencing life's bounty of sensual pleasures may be seen as a gift of being alive.

We oft heard the phrase "To each, his own." Exploring one's own metaphysical beliefs has immensely practical implications. Recognizing this truth will help us understand the most fascinating creature in the universe—ourselves.

On a personal basis, it is important that we understand how powerfully our beliefs and attitudes color the nature and quality of our lives. Do we see ourselves as victims of life's random absurdity? Or do we view painful and difficult circumstances as opportunities for spiritual growth and evolution?

Whether we see the glass as half empty or half full may very well determine not only the level of satisfaction in our lives but our physical health as well. When we recognize that our physical bodies are one component of a larger whole including mind and spirit, we cannot help but view life and its challenges from a greater perspective. We become less obsessed with the material world when we understand that it is not the totality of reality.

This book looks at healing in the broader context and defines it as that which makes us whole. It honors any and all activities and choices that make us more aware, knowledgeable, caring, compassionate, loving, and joyful.

Studying can be healing, helping others can be healing, learning can be healing, teaching can be healing. Pain can be a source of healing. We can learn more from difficult lessons than easy ones. Helping others overcome their own fears and challenges is healing. Sharing thoughts and feelings with others, especially in times of suffering and transformation, is a divine aspect of the healing process.

COME WITH ME ...

This book is organized to take you on a quest. I begin by sharing my own personal metaphysical journey. By sharing, I want you to see that even hard-core skeptics can experience a transformation when they open their minds to a new reality. In this book I seek to promote a perspective that integrates the lessons of science and spirituality into a new way of being, one that helps you find joy, peace, and healing in this world.

In this book, you will discover how to understand your own mind and how it creates your reality. And you will

- Learn the anatomy of how you formulate your beliefs.
- Validate your spiritual journey and personal experiences, and trust your gut feelings about others.
- Discover why fear of the unknown can paralyze your minds and freeze your actions.
- Find out how to counteract fear of the unknown with a deeper awareness.
- Learn to create a new reality for yourself at any time.
- Manage sadness and the dark side of feelings by seeing pain and suffering through new eyes.
- Overcome the fear of death and dying.
- Discover how healing yourself contributes to the healing of the world.
- Master ways to interpret life as a great mystery that can be explored with a skeptical open mind that balances feeling with knowledge, and belief with practicality.

Throughout this book, I offer many prescriptions for living. The most important one is: Be open-minded, yet retain a skeptical outlook. These are not contradictory points of view at all. With the assistance of multiple experts and points of view, we are all capable of evaluating truth for ourselves. This applies to deeply philosophical and religious beliefs, as well as the practical aspects of our approaches to health care and healing. We must seek evidence and reason in our approach to living and be practical as well. We may never totally understand how the universe works (who does?), but we can evaluate how successful different strategies can be within the context of our own lives.

In the expanding field of complementary and alternative medicine, it is wise to be open minded yet skeptical. I give the same advice to my patients who embrace the more traditional approaches to health care as well.

Quite simply, whatever leads us to a sense of wholeness and peace, promotes within us a deep understanding that there is a purpose to our lives, and helps us conquer our own fears is a prescription worth filling.

I am here to share my own prescriptions for enriching our lives through the metaphysical journey. Self-awareness precedes self-healing, and it is my hope that readers will gather insights into creating a better life for themselves.

I firmly believe that each of us can benefit from regular Metaphysical Checkups, but these are not exams you will get in your doctor's office. They are *self*-exams. This book gives you the tools and insight to do it for yourself.

Part I

My Personal Journey

The healer does not "do" or "give" something to the healee; instead he helps him come home to the All, to the One, to the way of "unity" with the Universe, and in this meeting the healee becomes more complete and this in itself is healing. In Arthur Koestler's words, "there is no sharp dividing line between self-repair and self-realization."

—Lawrence LeShan

1

From Physician to Meta-Physician: My Personal Journey from Physician to Healer

I was trained to be a physician, not a healer.

That statement may seem confusing or self-contradictory. After all, aren't physicians by definition healers? On the contrary, my journey from physician to meta-physician has shown me that the terms *physician* and *healer* are not interchangeable at all. As a product of the traditional approach to medicine, the methods and attitudes I encountered led me to view the patient as a machine suffering from some mechanical failure. My purpose was to be the best diagnostician possible, to identify the defective organ or organ system, with the goal of prescribing the appropriate tests and subsequent medication to treat and hopefully cure the patient. In all fairness, this may not have been the stated intention of my professors and mentors, but the system as it existed led inexorably to such an attitude and impression.

Of course, on some level I was aware that the patient had other dimensions to his or her being, including personal, emotional, and spiritual sides. Yet rarely in all my medical training did any of these factors rise to the level of my conscious awareness. It has only been within the last few years of my medical career that I have come to the profound realization that I have not been a healer at all. To *heal* means to "make whole" and, in the process of becoming aware, I changed. The Greek prefix *meta* signifies transformation—I became a meta-physician.

That epiphany required a major transformation in my spiritual perspective on life. As a product of the baby boomer generation, I had followed the path that embraced science as the ultimate arbiter of truth. Finding no evidence of God in the heavens, I declared science the winner. Although I managed the arduous trek through medical school, residency, and fellowship, in hindsight, I began my metaphysical quest in my undergraduate years with a degree in religious studies. Perhaps such a choice seemed inconsistent with my basic agnosticism and extreme skepticism. Yet it offered a broad humanities approach to this universal human endeavor. In retrospect, I suspect it was part of a larger plan for me—one that lay hidden for decades.

My career in medicine should have put to rest any consideration of spiritual exploration. Yet when I turned 50, something interrupted my straight-line atheism—the study of Kabbalah. It was not the study of the material itself that began to chip away at my shell of disbelief—it was ordinary and sincere people, enticed by my study of Kabbalah, who began to reveal to me deeply personal spiritual experiences. These experiences had a profound and life-altering effect upon my consciousness and contributed greatly to a profound change in my attitudes and beliefs regarding the nature of reality. There was something so compelling in those personal anecdotes that I could not ignore their metaphysical implications. I classified these mystical stories into near-death experiences, after-death communications, reincarnation memories, and medium and psychic experiences. These stories have become my evidence for a higher, more powerful spiritual reality. I soon came to realize that my own encounters with the paranormal were the tip of an iceberg that was available to all.

This diversion from my orthodox practice of gastroenterology seemed at first to offer me some amusing, if not curious glimpses of an unknown and unexplored universe. Intrigued, it stimulated me to explore a wide array of metaphysical, mystical, and spiritual literature and to recognize a fascinating pattern, a common thread that provided fuel for my journey of inquiry. At the same time, I began to revisit contemporary science: quantum theory, molecular biology, origin of life, and mind and consciousness studies. To my amazement, I began to see correspondences between all my studies. Science was not capable of debunking the personal spiritual stories I'd heard. Rather, science was deeply mired in its own metaphysical conundrum—it was unable to put back the pieces of the mechanical universe it had so vigorously defended for the past four hundred years. I began to see for the first time that science was engaged in its own process of evolving toward greater knowledge. It was a powerful force for uncovering the mysteries of the cosmos, yet it remained incomplete. Perhaps the mystics were on to something profound—spirit had not been banished from the cosmos after all.

In hindsight, I can hardly believe that I did not foresee the direction of my journey. My metaphysical quest began to turn, as if by its own will, back to my practice of medicine. Healing became the ultimate reason for my own personal journey; along the way I discovered it could possibly be the mission of all living beings as well. I began to truly see myself as a healer and not just as a physician. It became clear that the mind, body, and spirit could no longer be separated. Each needed to be addressed. For the first time I understood what (w)holism really meant. Even the distinction between healer and healee became blurred because the giving is equal to the receiving.

What had been my profession alone became much more. When I would attempt to reach out to another being, I began to feel a joy that cannot be put in words. Healing became more than an occupation. It became an attitude, a perspective, and an underlying paradigm for living.

STEPPING ONTO THE SPIRITUAL PATH

"How did you get into all of this?"

"Where did you decide to pursue metaphysics . . . this spiritual stuff you always talk and write about?"

"And when did you become interested in holistic healing?"

I've been responding to these questions for a long time, not only to the students in my Brookdale College classes on Contemporary Metaphysics but to family members, old friends, medical associates, and people I meet socially. And quite frankly, I have felt those questions, unexpressed but palpably present, from new acquaintances, fellow physicians, and patients as well. Perhaps the only one not surprised by these developments was me.

My resume of training and professional activities would have revealed no hint of such a metaphysical bent. My credentials, practice methods, hospital activities were clearly mainstream. I graduated from Albert Einstein College of Medicine, received my Internal Medicine training at Montefiore Hospital and Medical Center in the Bronx, and followed with my gastroenterology fellowship at Mount Sinai Medical Center in New York City. I was board certified in both, and had even served on the hospital executive board and two terms as President of the Medical Staff of Raritan Bay Medical Center. I've had an otherwise satisfying and "successful" practice in gastroenterology for nearly thirty years. I have complained with my colleagues over the malpractice fiasco, increasing costs of running a practice, the obscene profits of insurance companies at the expense of physicians and patients, and the overall decline of a once great profession.

However, at an age when many of my contemporaries are pondering how and when to retire, or where to buy that condo in Florida, I'm writing this book— and thinking about the nature of reality. I can't be sure what my colleagues and contemporaries think about my present interests. I hope that they respect the fact that I have always taken my duties and responsibilities to practice medicine with sincerity and diligence. I regard myself as an open-minded skeptic and regard the healing claims of traditional and alternative therapies to be equally suspect. Evidence needs to be sought in all forms of healing. But when it is present, it must not be ignored, regardless of its source. One point is clear to me—my metaphysical journey is much more than a self-indulgent exercise. I truly regard it as the source of my evolving understanding of the nature of reality, of my own life and those around me, and the nature of healing itself.

META-PHYSICIAN IN TRAINING?

Curiosity has been my constant companion throughout my life, from my earliest memories on. I was the product of a family of loving and supportive parents. As simple as that sentence might be, I do not take for granted the sense of calm, love, and serenity that was my foundation. I have come to realize how precious that beginning truly was. I recall an otherwise ordinary but fulfilling suburban childhood. Well behaved and essentially a conformist, I doubt that there were many *overt* signs that I might get "metaphysical" as I got older.

Although perhaps the signs were there, in embryonic form: I was fascinated by astronomy, microscopic organisms, dinosaurs, and fossils. I seemed to recall reading "strange but true" books with bizarre examples of natural phenomena. The abominable snowman, monitor lizards, and giant squids were the stuff of both fiction and nonfiction for me. Cartoons and comics provided me with a picture of early man that I assumed to be true. Fred Flintstone and Barney Rubble had dinosaurs as pets. Movies showed cavemen battling Tyrannosaurus Rex and a flying Pterodactyl. When I subsequently learned that dinosaurs had gone extinct millions of years before humans, I found myself in a state of existential shock. It was a feeling of both confusion and excitement. I was clearly unaware of the term *cognitive dissonance* (the sudden awareness that one's previous beliefs might be incorrect) but I knew that I had received a jolt to my view of reality. It was a sign to me that I should not automatically accept as truth everything that was offered as such. It was an exciting feeling of a new insight, a personal discovery that might just change the way I would look at the world around me. It was a feeling that would return to me in spades years later.

And, furthermore, if I could have been wrong about that—what was next? Perhaps those Bible stories about Adam, Eve, and God were equally wrong? My mother, who was always present and available, would often have to listen to my "discoveries" about nature, microscopic protozoa, fossils found in the backyard, and any variety of unusual facts about the natural world. I knew that she really wasn't as excited as I was, but still she seemed to listen attentively, while probably wondering where I came from. Sadly, she passed away as I was writing this book. For years prior, she suffered from a slowly progressive memory loss (a variant of Alzheimer's dementia). I always made it a point to relate some of the spiritual experiences I was writing about to both my parents. I was trying to offer them some sense of peace about what came after life. One day, toward the end of my mother's life, I shared a story about reincarnation. In one of her more lucid moments, she plainly stated, "Steve was always a weird kid." I laughed out loud. It was an episode of spontaneously revealed truth. It was a poignant moment for me, one that was filled with humor and sadness. When I was young and formulating my view of the world, she would have never expressed her true feelings or opinions about the things I shared with her. Now, nearing the end of her life, the veils were lowered, and she could reveal her true thoughts about the strange thread that weaved its way through her otherwise ordinary child.

Religion was a subject that I had always found interesting, especially the notion that one could "be Jewish" without necessarily being religious. For me, being born into the Jewish faith was as much a historical and ethnic identity and it was one that I was proud of. But I felt no strong spiritual connection to Judaism, or any other religion for that matter. Although I participated in the cultural rituals—Passover, high holidays—I stayed clear of the religious aspects.

My feeling was: Science supplied all the truth that anyone needed to know about the natural world. Religion was a human invention, a necessary sanctuary against the unexplained, unwelcome chaos of existence. That made perfect sense to me. In the absence of any evidence to the contrary, I had no choice but to doubt the existence of God, the soul, or any notion of life after death. I definitely dwelled in a belief system somewhere between atheist and agnostic, with a strong dose of existentialism for an added kick.

"SO, YOU WANT TO BE A RABBI?"

I recall frequently explaining to people why I chose to major in Religious Studies in my undergraduate days at Franklin and Marshall College in Lancaster, Pennsylvania. Many people assumed I wanted to become a rabbi. The truth was quite simple: I found the study of religion completely fascinating! Religion was a universal human experience, practiced in all cultures, across all continents, throughout all of human history. I was the outsider looking in. For me it was like studying anthropology, sociology, or psychology. I was not seeking to resolve my inner metaphysical turmoil, nor was I seeking a new spiritual platform. These were simply intellectually stimulating subjects, taught by open-minded, highly intelligent professors, who could educate and enlighten me about this seemingly universal human phenomenon.

Another reason for my excitement was my studies: I finally had an opportunity to read the New Testament, the basis of Christianity and, with it, much of Western Civilization. The course materials merely convinced me further that religion was a human invention. To my mind, none of it reflected anything I recognized as "higher truths." One of my favorite professors, Bradley Dewey, Ph.D., was an expert on the Danish theologian and philosopher Soren Kierkegaard. He would describe the concept of the *leap of faith*, a rejection of logic and reason in pursuit of the Divine that was needed to attain a state of religious belief.

I could understand what *belief* meant. It was our personal opinion or conclusion about something, and represented the sum total of all our feelings and thoughts. But why abandon reason and evidence in this process of belief? I was certainly able to live with the mystery of existence. It would be absurd to think that man could possibly understand everything. Yet I also believed that there must be more to it than "just have faith." There had to be *evidence*! There had to be some path by which my reason could lead me down the path to the truth. My inner skeptic screamed out: Why should I have to abandon my mind, my powers of reason, to find God?

At this juncture, it was the late sixties and early seventies, times of political, intellectual, and spiritual upheaval in this country. While traditional religions were defending themselves against the claims of atheists that "God Is Dead," alternative and Eastern religious practices were having an impact on the college generation and American culture as well. None of this appealed to me. I felt no spiritual impulse or attraction to any of it. I regarded the Hare Krishna movement and other Eastern imports as rather silly and irrelevant.

THE ROAD TAKEN

Medical school admission—it was the Gold Medal for many young students of my generation. An M.D. was regarded a key to financial and material success. However, believe it or not, I truly didn't see it that way. I was not one of those students who had always dreamed of becoming a doctor. Unsure of a career choice,

I was advised by my mother to try pre-med courses as an alternative to being drafted in the ongoing conflict in Vietnam. Once I started on this path, there was no turning back. In hindsight, a door opened for me, and I entered. As events unfolded, I felt privileged to be able to pursue a time-honored and noble profession. In fact, I was rather shocked that I had been admitted to medical school at all. I assumed that a Religious Studies major would put me at a disadvantage because I was competing with math–science all-stars. Fortunately, the admissions directors at several schools saw my different background as potentially of interest—and I got in.

By that point in time, I had put my fascination with the religious impulse aside. I might have pursued an academic career in teaching or publishing. But I didn't. It became the road *not taken*—a seductive, vaguely forbidden pathway that remained buried in my consciousness for the years that followed. I was headed for a more conventional career, one that offered stability and security.

Science was king and I had to dig into the task at hand. I recall studying and memorizing large quantities of information. There was little patient contact the first year and a half of medical school, and the work was understandably tedious.

If I had entered my training with some vague hope that I would eventually be able to offer compassion and dedication to my fellow human beings, it was gradually being drained away by the process itself. There were opportunities to escape the grind at times, but this precious free time was devoted to partying and going out. I could not summon the energy, interest, or will to explore the metaphysical universe.

There was a fraternity-like attitude toward medical education at the time, one that most assuredly carried over into residency. There was little time for personal reflection or metaphysical discussions about the nature of reality back then. We were all "under the gun" to study and perform on examinations. Physically and emotionally drained, these were not the conditions by which one evolves into a caring and compassionate healer.

The long hours, lack of sleep, and competitive pressure to perform were oftentimes overwhelming. Like rites of passage, we were expected to suffer in order to gain admittance to the tribe.

Never once during all my years of medical school, residency, and fellowship did I hear the term *healing* used. I heard let's "diagnose," "treat," "manage," even "cure" the patient—as if they were nothing more than mannequins with labels that indicate which disease they are. I believe that true healing, literally "to make whole," requires an intimate human connection. Sadly, my understanding of the nature of healing was not derived from my period of training. It was only after many years of practice, and my venture into metaphysics, that this became clear to me. Fortunately, contemporary medical educators have made attempts to address these issues. Although far from perfect, their efforts should be applauded. Over time, I began to understand healing at a deeply metaphysical level: that it is the attainment, by each individual soul, of its highest potential. With this understanding, it became clear to me that no one can totally heal another. A physician who is aware of all aspects of mind, body and spirit can educate the patient as well as guide, advise and prescribe.

Our physical bodies possess miraculous abilities to repair and regenerate themselves. Our immune system is in a constant state of awareness and activity. Eventually I would become aware that healing truly meant "to make whole" and that this could not be achieved without considering the patient's emotional and spiritual aspects.

MY FIRST TIME

While in medical school I met and married Ardith, a beautiful, loving woman who has remained my wife and partner since 1973. Together we've raised two amazing children. She has been there to temper some of my recent enthusiasm. In hindsight, however, she was there when we had our first paranormal experience. We were dating and she brought out a Ouija board. I had never seen one before. Ardith described having played with one in her youth with another friend and received some "strange" readings.

We had our own session that night. It was a fascinating experience with paranormal readings, movements, and messages that I cannot rationally explain. The plastic planchette literally flew across the board, spelling out names and dates. It seemed that a male and a female were trying to "communicate" with us. Each described how and when they died. Most bizarre of all was the male described the date and location of his death as the Sudetenland, in 1939. We were not quite sure where this was. Was this Europe or Africa? We discovered that it was a part of Czechoslovakia that Hitler entered in the months leading up to World War II. Many were killed during this period.

It was a chilling experience—one that challenged my rational thought processes. There was a part of me that wanted to doubt and disbelieve it, yet I knew that it was real, that we were not manipulating the results, that it was happening to the two of us, and that there was no one else physically in the room. It was not coming from our subconscious minds, yet it could not be explained. It was another moment of *cognitive dissonance*, an experience that challenged my sense of reality. It remains unexplained to me—to this day. Like many who have had similar experiences, I didn't know what to do with it. It didn't fit into my scientific paradigm. It certainly was not something I would mention to my medical colleagues. Interesting, I later discovered that something similar occurred to Dr. Stephen E. Braude, Ph.D., who subsequently wrote several books presenting evidence for life after death. He still refers to his own Ouija experience as an unexplained but significant impetus to his eventual study of the field. He could never adequately explain what he had experienced that day, but he never forgot it and ultimately retained its impact as motivation for his own metaphysical journey.

So what does anyone do with such an experience? It suggested a moment of cosmic uncertainty to me. I could deny that something strange, paranormal had occurred. Yet I couldn't explain exactly what it meant. It clashed with my rational and empirical atheism. I had no choice but to file it away in the deepest recesses of my mind—in the folder marked "mystery." This mental file of the unknown remained locked away for many years and with it, my inner metaphysical quest.

KABBALAH 101—THE EARLY ENCOUNTER

During the winter of 1995, I decided to attend a series of lectures by an Orthodox Rabbi, given at the home of a member of our synagogue. My innate spiritual curiosity was rekindled. My background in religious studies, along with casual reading over the years, had provided me with an awareness of Kabbalah. From what I knew, it was a mystical form of Judaism, traditionally reserved for men over age 40 that were very learned in the rituals and teachings of their faith.

This was before Kabbalah was *hot*, and before it was part of the mainstream public's awareness. Madonna and other celebrities were just quietly beginning their own explorations. Kabbalah was still pretty much in the closet. Looking back at my first experience, I felt Kabbalah could have stayed in the closet! The first lecture I attended bordered between dull and ridiculous. It was uninspiring and confusing.

The Rabbi was a follower of the Ultra-orthodox Chabad-Lubavitch branch of Chassidic Judaism and he was, oddly enough, lecturing to a group of far less religious Jews. When asked why he was even making the effort to reach Jews who barely considered themselves Jewish he said: "Because the answers have all been revealed and the time is right to share them with the world." The implication was that it was time to reveal the information to the masses in order to facilitate the coming of the Messiah. This was *way* too religious for me!

At the same time, I found it curious that he was talking about subjects that seemed so out of place for a rabbi. For example, he suggested one could easily find a parking space simply by meditating on it. He also said he'd been receiving Kabbalah teachings on a nightly basis for an entire year from his mentor, Rabbi Horowitz —who happened to be dead. The discussion of paranormal phenomenon did not stop there. I was not only unimpressed by these tales, I was annoyed. I felt like walking out. Almost everything he said seemed so preposterous to me. I wondered: "What was a rabbi doing speaking about bogus New Age stuff, anyway?"

There was another story that seemed very wacky to me at the time. It concerned a late-night library session, during which time, according to this Rabbi, his esteemed mentor seemed to, as he put it, "float into the library, very smooth, like a wizard." He was asked by his spiritual mentor if he wanted to reach his highest destiny, and when he said "yes," he was told: "Then you must become a Master of Free Will. You can think about ideas as paintings in a gallery. Look at them, think about them, take them home and hang them in your home. You can choose what you want to believe and it will become your reality."

That was just about enough for me. It sounded like a scene out of *Fiddler on the Roof* and frankly, it was like a bad night at the theater. My first exposure to

Kabbalah was very odd and it left me feeling rather disappointed. Wasn't this the mystical, secretive aspect of Judaism, for so long kept hidden from the majority of Jews? Could this have been all there was to it? Despite my disappointment, I perceived some small kernel of fascination.

No one was more surprised when, three years later, I would be reintroduced to Kabbalistic teachings and it would change my life for the better and enrich me in ways that I would have never imagined. It was a perfect demonstration to me that events occur in our lives at a particular time, for a particular reason. Unless all factors are in proper alignment, there may be little gained from the encounter. Fortunately, I had kept the tapes from those earlier classes. As I listened to them again I was astounded. I now understood the message that was being delivered. We can choose what we want to believe, and our choices affect our experience of everyday living. Interestingly, I also came across the concept of "choosing what you want to believe" from a rather unlikely source—Albert Einstein. Amazed as I was that a man of science could express those sentiments, he seemed to back up what the Rabbi had shared.

Several years later, I began to understand that the deeply human preoccupation with the arts had metaphysical implications as well. We are creative beings whose minds can choose how we interpret the universe, choose our personal view of reality, and choose the picture we live in. This is a concept that would help me enhance my understanding of the mind–body–spirit connection in a deeply profound way. It would change me, and would enhance the way I would practice medicine.

I discovered a Kabbalah Centre that had opened in Manhattan and, despite my less than fantastic first impression, I was curious enough to attend a series of classes for nearly a year. By then, Kabbalah had been formatted for a New Age–seeking public and Madonna's name was more openly associated with it. To be honest, the lectures and methods of the Centre itself were wildly appealing to many students of a variety of backgrounds. But I found them a bit predigested. Nevertheless, they did motivate me to seek the nearest Barnes & Noble bookstore and begin my own explorations. A new door had opened for me and I gladly stepped across the threshold.

KABBALAH 102–SPIRITUAL JUDAISM

One of my most startling discoveries was that Judaism has such a strong spiritual and mystical tradition and it is embodied in Kabbalistic teachings. This seems like a strange statement to make, especially from someone who was raised with a typical Jewish education, followed by an undergraduate exposure to religious studies. But much of what I learned through Kabbalah simply had not been part of my culturally Jewish upbringing.

Meditation is a Jewish concept? Karma is a Jewish concept? Reincarnation is a Jewish concept? The concept of the soul is Jewish? Through the Kabbalistic perspective the answer to all of these questions was a resounding *yes*! Why hadn't I been aware of this? And furthermore, why would the vast majority of contemporary Jews still not believe it? The fact that this tradition had been sidetracked, nearly eradicated from much of Western European and American Judaism, is an entire book in itself. In short, Jews believed that to present a more "acceptable" face to the Christian world, they needed to jettison that which was different—clothes, dietary habits, and mysticism. Only the Orthodox groups, the Hasidic movement, joyously retained and expanded the mysticism of Kabbalah.

I began to see fascinating correspondences between Kabbalah and more Eastern belief systems: Buddhism, Hinduism, and Sufism (which is the mystical aspect of Islam). It seems as if there was no coincidence that a large number of "Western" Buddhists, and Hindus, were born Jews. The Dalai Lama himself was more than aware of this fact. Ironically, these Jews were seeking a deeper spirituality from sources outside of their own tradition, mainly because they were unaware of Kabbalah. They did not know it was all there, in their own religion. I read a fascinating book, *The Jew in the Lotus,* which chronicled the visit of American Jews to the Dalai Lama. There were fascinating parallels between such divergent religious philosophies. Many of the books I was finding were written by Rabbis, male and female, who had returned to Judaism after long excursions into the teachings of these Eastern theologies. They found their spiritual home in the rediscovered teachings of Kabbalah. I was finding this return home rather enticing as well.

TRUTH IS ONE, PEOPLE CALL IT BY DIFFERENT NAMES

In my earlier days I had developed a belief that all religious beliefs were fantasy—therefore it mattered little what anyone believed. But as I began to reclaim my metaphysical quest I began to realize there had to be, ultimately, one truth. I had still to be convinced that there was any reality to the claims of religion (the institution of) or spirituality (the belief in a Spirit or God, the soul, life after death). If there is one physics, one biology, one chemistry, one cosmology, and so on, then there can be but one metaphysical truth about the domain of spirit, soul, and divinity.

All religions, therefore, being different from one another to a certain degree, are most likely not completely "correct." How could they be? But of course, we human beings respond with our typical defensiveness and reactivity: "No, you are wrong! My religion is correct! The others are blasphemy! If you go against my religion, you are evil, or an infidel. Non-belief is the devil's design!"

Acknowledging that religions are human interpretations of divinity, I believe we should recognize that each has unique historical, political, and historical roots, that they are all *optional* paths to the one truth. It is here that I stepped back from the study of religion and came to understand the concept of spirituality for the first time. Religion is institutionalized spirituality. Spirituality is the mystical core of all religion. It is the overlay of history, ritual, practices, and politics that produces the dramatic and visible differences between the world's religions.

A study of the writings and experiences of the mystics of each religion, however, reveals a surprising similarity. "All mystics come from the same country, speak the same language," said philosopher and theologian Louis Claude de St. Martin. Philosopher C.D. Broad concurred: "The similarities between the statements of mystics all the world over seems to be a really significant fact." I began to focus on the spiritual core of these differing belief systems. This could in theory also be a pathway toward reducing the age-old animosities that serve as the source of so much suffering and hatred in our contemporary world. The insight that the most spiritually gifted human beings have encountered the divine in similar ways should offer us all hope for a more peaceful coexistence. Despite my belief that there was One Ultimate Truth, I acknowledged that certain images, metaphors, and explanations would resonate with me more than others. Kabbalah continued to offer them.

CREATION METAPHORS: A SHATTERED UNIVERSE AND HUMANITY AS HEALER

Even after studying Kabbalah in earnest, my metaphysical journey was at a crossroads. I still had no evidence by which to abandon my hard-core skeptical agnosticism. Still, there was something appealing to me about the Kabbalistic metaphysical position. Rabbi Isaac Luria, the sixteenth-century mystic from Safed, Israel, offered a fascinating Kabbalistic reinterpretation of the creation myth, in which he stated we inhabit a divinely inspired, but imperfect universe. He postulated that the imperfection is the consequence of shattered vessels and that the entire world, both inanimate and animate, rock and humanity, were secret repositories of Holy Sparks. By this interpretation, humanity assumed an enormous role: to act as co-Creator, and to recognize and liberate the divine sparks that resided within all matter.

Although I was far from convinced that this was little more than pure mythology, the notion that humanity's role in the universe was crucial for the spiritual evolution of all of creation was appealing to me. If I was to accept any spiritual system it would have to be one that assumed individuals personally responsible for their actions and that would allow humanity a significant role in the way the universe unfolded. I could not personally relate to a belief system in which humankind's deeds could be "forgiven" through confession or faith alone, or that another being, physical or spiritual, could absolve anyone else of responsibility for one's actions.

Karma, too, seemed to make sense to me. It placed the responsibility for one's actions squarely where they belonged, on the individuals themselves. The ultimate purpose for this accounting of actions was not for punishment but for learning and spiritual evolution. The possibility of reincarnation, of multiple lifetimes, was a necessary component of the karmic system. Kabbalah described such a system, one in which each lifetime represented an opportunity to choose the path toward spiritual evolution.

The Kabbalistic concept for humanity's role in the entire metaphysical system repair is *tikkun*. It means to repair, fix, or heal. The notion was that to repair or heal our souls, we must heal the world. This makes humankind's social responsibilities a spiritual endeavor as well. This was an extraordinary concept to me: Healing as correction . . . healing as learning . . . healing as personal growth . . . healing as spiritual, moral, and mental evolution. This was much bigger than the limited perspective of one individual's physical body. In this expanded sense, healing became nothing less than the goal of human existence—our purpose for being. Aha! Finally, I seemed to have at least one answer to the question "Why are we here?" It was a notion of healing that resonated with me, one that would become the basis for my own metaphysical platform.

INTRODUCING THE "GOOD WITCH"

Something quite dramatic happened to me during the time I was attending Kabbalah classes in 1998. I became acquainted with someone I considered a "Good Witch." This woman—I'll call her Jen—would hate the label but it is so fitting I cannot resist. One early morning, on hospital rounds, I had a conversation with a nurse on duty, someone I had known for several years. In response to the typical question "What's new?" I mentioned my study of Kabbalah and explained what it was about—Jewish Mysticism. Her immediate response: "You must speak with Jen . . . she's had 'experiences'!"

My curiosity was definitely aroused. Jen and I had never spoken to each other on a personal basis, and it became clear that she was quite shy and hesitant by nature; in addition, she was quite reluctant about speaking with me about these experiences. She would not chat at the hospital, in public, and quietly asked me to call her later at home. I did. I explained that I had no unusual experiences of my own but that I was a student of religion, of Kabbalah, and was interested in the study of spirituality and mysticism. I had once read a book about the near-death experience (NDE) and even had a patient who described her own experience to me. That was the extent of what I knew.

I convinced Jen that I would take what she said seriously. She slowly began to reveal a lifetime of strange paranormal encounters. She said as a child she always *knew* who in her family would die before they passed. She always *knew* who was on the phone before it was picked up. She *saw* departed relatives in her home. She was terribly distressed and frightened by these premonitions and experiences. When she told her mother, the reaction was not one of surprise. Apparently, this *ability* did run in the family. She was told merely to keep quiet about it—that people wouldn't understand.

Jen revealed an especially painful moment from her teenage years. Her mother had made a birthday party for her and she had quite a few friends and acquaintances over her house. Several of her friends knew about her ability and one said, "Jen, guess what my Mom got you. . . . I don't really know myself." Jen proceeded to describe a yellow bathrobe with white flowers. When she opened the wrapping paper, there it was. One of the boys screamed out, "Oooh, you're a witch." The shy teenager was mortified. This label was exactly what she did not want to hear. This fear about being mocked has persisted in Jen. And it was this reluctance to discuss her strange abilities that drew me in further. I could see she had nothing to gain by fabricating any of this. In fact, the situation was precisely the opposite—she feared that I, too, would regard her as bizarre, or worse.

Over the next several months Jen would reveal a great deal more about her experiences. She slowly began to trust that I took her seriously. She revealed mostly frightening premonitions: about a fire at her uncle's factory before it occurred, a series of high-profile airplane crashes as well. She was tortured by these insights for which she could do nothing. She sought help from a priest, as well as a minister. She was told that Joseph in the Bible had the same kind of gift from God. That didn't help Jen. She was clearly suffering.

One of the most painful premonitions for her occurred shortly after she met her husband. He was somewhat put off by her abilities. One day while driving in the car he bluntly called out to her, "So if you know everything, how old will I be when I die." She immediately "knew" that he would not reach his fortieth birthday. The pain was immense for her. She tried to hide this from him. Unfortunately, she was right once more—about seven years later he contracted lymphoma and died when he was 39.

For several years Jen would reluctantly and privately report to me new and frightening experiences. I saw her after the tragedy of 9/11. She knew what I wanted to hear. She pulled me aside and, in hushed tones, told me that on September 10, she was washing her breakfast dishes when she felt an explosion in her chest and saw the Twin Towers. She dropped to her knees and began sobbing, as well as praying. Approximately fifteen minutes later, a second explosion. The times were identical to those that occurred the following day. She was sick for the twenty-four hours preceding the actual event. They occurred as she "saw" them.

As if that wasn't enough, Jen said to me one day, "I saw another one—there will be another horrible plane crash." I quickly asked her to tell me as much as possible about what she saw. "It's not a jumbo jet, it has a nose like a Lear Jet and I'm on the plane when it goes down." No mention of a jet crash occurred in the news for nearly a week. I had nearly forgotten about her prediction—until it happened—the infamous crash of a Concorde jet—which led to the demise of the entire Concorde line. The next morning her eyes were heavy and bloodshot. "That was it," she said.

My communication with Jen was the beginning of what has become a totally fascinating collection of personal experiences that have become the fuel for my metaphysical journey. Even before it was crystal clear to me that Jen was telling the absolute truth, and that there was absolutely no reason for her to lie or exaggerate or fabricate any of it, *I got it*. This was her reality, and thus, it was real. For Jen, this ability was more of a curse than a gift. For me, it was a transformative experience and I am grateful that she allowed me into her world.

My fascination with Jen and her experiences led me to mention them (anonymously) to others around me—my office staff, friends, and acquaintances. What followed was even more amazing. Many of these people had experiences as well. Only when I probed did they begin to reveal these extraordinary experiences with spirituality and the paranormal.

OPENING THE METAPHYSICAL FLOODGATES

It was not my intention to expose Jen, or turn her compelling stories into entertainment, but I felt inspired to continue to speak about what she'd shared. I felt she had come into my life for a reason, as I had come into hers. What followed was even more amazing to me.

My office manager, Louise, is a woman for whom I had and continue to have enormous respect. Her response to hearing Jen's stories was a brief smile . . . and a knowing nod. "You mean you're not surprised?" I asked. "No, not at all," she said. "You see I've had quite a few of my own experiences."

I must have stood with my mouth open as she described her encounter with the "other side" in her home in Florida, which had a typical fenced-in patio. "One evening I 'saw' two elderly gentlemen walk right into my porch through one side of the closed area," she relayed. "They were speaking to each other and seemed not to notice me at all. I can still recall the clothes, shirt, pants and shoes that each wore. They moved slowly and I could see through them. Then they faded away. I knew that I had seen two ghosts. What's more, I spoke to one of the neighbors who had lived in the area for many years before we moved in. They recalled that our home had been used as an illegal home for elderly men—several had died there before they closed down the activities there."

I was astounded. Here was a rational, intelligent, and down-to-earth woman whom I had known and respected for years. She was not someone whom I would have pegged for having paranormal experiences. It made me wonder, who did I expect these people to be? Over the succeeding years, I have learned that there is no "typical" person. These experiences occur to people of all backgrounds and all walks of life. So, why not me? Ah . . . a question I have also pondered. Why should someone be as interested in these phenomena as I am and not have had their own experience?

I recall reading that the great psychologist, physician, and intellectual William James, cofounder of the American Society of Psychical Research, expressed his own disappointment in not having his own experiences. Perhaps there is a role for us—those with "mystic envy." Perhaps, by being outsiders we can evaluate and discuss what happens to others with more objectivity.

THE PURPLE DRESS WITH YELLOW POLKA DOTS

Was it pure chance or coincidence that another one of my employees happened to overhear Louise's story and felt compelled to share her own? Brenda, also, seemed an unlikely storyteller. She was about my age, professional, very pleasant, and *totally* down to earth. She shared the following experience that has clearly been a part of her consciousness since childhood.

> I can never forget this one particular day: I was nine years old and had just gotten home from school when my mother asked me to go upstairs and comfort my dad. She told me that my uncle Joe, his brother, had died suddenly. I walked up the stairs and was about to enter his bedroom when I saw through the partially opened door my father lying across the bed and sobbing. An elderly woman with grey hair was stroking his head and shoulders and saying, "Don't worry Johnny, Joey is alright. You'll be with him soon." I didn't know who the old lady was but I recall that she was wearing a purple dress with yellow polka dots. I was surprised to hear anyone call my dad Johnny—no one ever did. I walked back downstairs and explained to my mother that there was an old lady with Dad in the bedroom. She said, "there's no one else here in the house." When I described the dress, she turned pale. I later found out that I had described my grandmother, who had died before I was born and was buried in that dress. Not only that, but my father died suddenly three months later.

I was truly amazed by this story as well. My skeptical side tried to analyze it—was there any motivation to make up or embellish such a strange tale? But it also gave me chills—confirmation that she was telling the truth. Who would make up a story involving the death of his or her own uncle, grandmother, and father? The details involved were also phenomenally compelling. What did all this truly mean? Why are people privy to these moments and flashes of insight and intuition? How is it they can see dead relatives and somehow know the circumstances of death for others? I was being exposed to a reality that I had never, ever imagined was true.

I continued to withhold my judgment about what I was hearing. I just listened. More stories flooded into my life, and into my awareness. One of my physician partners, Bob, recalled seeing the ghost of his own grandfather in the pose of offering a toast in the kitchen—something he had done often in life. To him it was as real as if he were standing there in the flesh. There were so many other stories as well. As I opened to hearing them, and considering them, more and more people shared them, the best of these stories offered me an element of "new knowledge." They became the backbone of the confirmatory evidence that I was gathering and they helped me know and these were more than one person's wishful thinking or fantasy.

I was deeply engaged in an attempt to make some sense of what I was hearing. If there was a spiritual dimension to reality, how would that transform my view of the nature of reality? What were the metaphysical implications? I also intuitively knew that to become obsessed over these experiences was to miss the deeper message behind them—if there is a spiritual reality, how can I use this awareness to be a better healer as well as a more evolved human being?

THE GOLD STANDARD OF ALL TRUTH—SCIENCE

Back when I was studying at the Kabbalah Centre, I heard some scientific references that seemed odd to me. In classes, instructors spoke of the 99 percent of open space that comprised the universe. Only 1 percent is matter, they said. To my mind, this scientific fact seemed so misplaced in a course on spirituality. But it tantalized me to learn more.

As I scanned dozens of books on Kabbalah, and general spirituality, I was blown away by some of titles—*The Mind of God, The Tao of Physics, The Quantum Mind and Healing,* and so on. Up until then, I'd been unaware of the enormous amount of New Age literature—written by physicists and other scientists—that explored the relationship between contemporary science and spirituality. I eagerly began to dig in and to explore the reasons I had always regarded science and religion as incompatible metaphysical systems. To be honest, I believe I was just one of many Americans to whom it seemed logical that science and spirituality were contradictory, incompatible belief systems.

Everyone knew that science had disproved the claims of the creation of the universe and of life contained within the book of Genesis. No one in my professional or social circles seriously questioned Darwinian evolution. Everyone knew that the universe was a machine that could be clearly understood by the laws of physics. Everyone knew that it was only a matter of time before science would clarify all questions and put religion and spirituality out of business. . . . Or so I thought!

I was of the mindset that no intelligent scientist could possibly justify a spiritual reality. It seemed obvious to me that professional scientists would, by virtue of their own study and work, be atheists. Then I began to come across insights, statements, and quotes, like these from Albert Einstein:

> Everyone who is seriously involved in the pursuit of science becomes convinced that a spirit is manifest in the laws of the universe—a spirit vastly superior to man.

And

> Science without religion is lame. Religion without science is blind.

Why hadn't I even considered that scientists could believe, or at least conceive of, a higher intelligence? This was a far cry from science "proving" a higher metaphysical reality. I also came across statistics that 40 percent of scientists believed in the existence of God. True, this was far below the over 90 percent of typical Americans who believe in God. Still, 40 percent of scientists? My only assumption could be that for these individuals, science had not closed the door on spirituality.

I began to read about the history of the relationship between science and religion. Many brilliant theologians and thinkers from the twelfth century, including

Christian theologian Thomas Aquinas and the Jewish physician and philosopher Moses Maimonides, found no conflict between the two. Science, the study of the natural world, was seen to simply reveal the wisdom of God. Problems arose when science began to challenge the dogma of the Bible. Technology, through the telescope, revealed that the sun, not the earth, was the center of the known universe. The Church saw an acceptance of such blasphemy as just the beginning of the loss of faith in its teachings.

A number of brilliant scientists—including Copernicus, Galileo, Newton, Bacon and Kepler—uncovered the mathematical laws that led to an understanding of the universe as an intricate but comprehensible machine. Strangely, this seventeenth-century notion gradually percolated into the very fabric of the scholarly and intellectual atmosphere of Western civilization. The Enlightenment Period continued to struggle with this notion that the mind of man, the ability to reason, would soon reveal all the secrets of the universe.

The universe was a machine, one that could be totally understood by the mind of man. There was no mystery left to uncover. Nineteenth-century French cosmologist Marquis de la Place, upon being questioned by Napoleon as to why he didn't include the name of God in his description of the cosmos replied famously, "Sire, I have no need for that hypothesis!"

What followed during the rest of the nineteenth century was an ever-expanding list of scientific accomplishments: the internal combustion engine, telegraph, telephone, the horseless carriage, electromagnetism, measuring the speed of light—and on and on. Gone were the days when God could be found in the "gaps" in man's knowledge. As these gaps were evaporating, so was the need for "that hypothesis."

That was all true, wasn't it? Ironically, philosophy, source of all metaphysical speculation, was beginning to question the value of metaphysics. Its long association with the search for ultimate meaning was being rejected by a movement within philosophy known as Logical Positivism, which embraced the achievements of science as the ultimate and exclusive path toward truth. Logical Positivists considered the debate about the meaning of existence essentially fruitless, a waste of time.

One of the twentieth century's most well-known philosophers, Bertrand Russell, noted: "Science is what you know. Philosophy is what you don't know." If not yet—then eventually. After all, the powerful and undeniable success of the scientific endeavor only proved that the universe was comprehensible to the mind of man.

Of course this made perfect sense to me, but, why then would Einstein offer statements that invoked a higher intelligence? The grand man of scientific thought seemed to be indulging in metaphysical speculation. I found it strange but intriguing—scientists were resurrecting that which philosophers had discarded themselves—metaphysics.

The answer seemed to lay in the discoveries of both relativity and quantum theory in the early years of the twentieth century. I read about the bizarre nature of relativity theory and was fascinated: The faster one traveled, the slower time ran; time and space actually formed a new dimension called "space-time" in which all events, past, present and future where located and existed simultaneously. The most famous mathematical equation in science, $E = mc^2$, energy was equivalent to mass times the speed of light squared, seemed as incomprehensible as any Kabbalistic meditation. Energy and mass were actually two forms of the same "substance." They were theoretically interconvertible, one to the other. Perhaps science was discovering what philosophers and mystics had always proclaimed, that the universe itself was One.

Quantum theory was even more counterintuitive: subatomic particles could appear, disappear, and reappear almost magically from the quantum vacuum without an explanation for their existence in between. Even their eventual location would be based on probability equations. The attempt to measure a particle's momentum and location always resulted in a level of uncertainty. Measuring one variable would affect the result of the other. The results of experiments revealed that light was either a wave or a particle—depending on how the experiment was conducted and the act of observation itself.

Two linked subatomic particles once separated and shot across the universe in opposite directions, always "knew" what happened to its twin, and responded faster than the speed of light. Known as quantum entanglement or nonlocality, Einstein could never accept this notion of "spooky action at a distance." Yet after his death, the great man was proven wrong. The universe was more spooky than even Einstein wanted to believe.

The notion that probability ruled over exactitude was another concept that even Einstein could never accept. His famous line "God doesn't play with dice" reflected his disapproval with this position. But even that, too, would prove to be correct.

As I became more aware of these findings, I found my own metaphysical foundations sinking. I, too, had assumed that science had all the answers, or at least was on its way to doing so. The universe was clearly not a neatly organized, comprehensible machine. What other surprises awaited me?

Again, I was amazed. Quantum physicists were expressing their absolute dismay. Paradox, counterintuitive findings, absolute uncertainty, and mystery seemed to be the metaphysical message of their experiments. Scientists were questioning their own sanity at times. Rather than revealing a universe that fit our mind's eye—the opposite seemed to be the case.

Recent discoveries now reveal that the entire physical universe of atoms, matter, planets, stars, and galaxies represent only 4 percent of the mass that exists. The rest is composed of dark matter and dark energy, and no one is quite sure what they are! Science was revealing a universe far more complex, less comprehensible than anyone knew how to handle.

It was understandable, therefore, that scientists were venturing into metaphysics to explain what they were uncovering about the universe. Some were comparing Eastern mysticism with their findings, others Western mysticism and

Kabbalah. Psychologist Lawrence LeShan wrote about physicists, mystics, and mediums and proposed that each had to enter another state of consciousness in order to comprehend their own experiences. Philosopher Ken Wilber likewise observed that contemporary scientists were writing like mystics.

Scientists are drawn to their profession because of the desire to discover reality and their absolute conviction that the truth will be revealed by their actions. They chose to investigate, experiment, and theorize in order to understand. Their beloved science was, in some ways, letting them down. They knew that quantum theory and relativity theory were correct because they could use their equations to advance not only science but modern computer and household technology. Computer chips, transistors, and lasers were all born of quantum theory. Scientists just couldn't explain it to others or even to themselves in old-fashioned, commonsense ways. The universe was not necessarily telling them that mysticism or spirituality was the path to metaphysical truth—but it was not eliminating this possibility either.

FINDING MY PLACE IN THE UNIVERSE

I was tremendously energized by my exposure to these subjects. It seemed as if three separate pathways were converging within my consciousness:

1. Kabbalistic mysticism
2. The spiritual and paranormal experiences I was hearing
3. Contemporary scientific thought.

My challenge was to use all this input, and all these aspects, to make sense of the nature of reality and perhaps lead me along a path of personal exploration and a more comprehensive notion of healing. To me it was becoming increasingly clear that all thinking human beings yearn to make sense of the world around them. We are all, therefore, meta-physicians. But by merging these three aspects of awareness, I was being transformed as a physician as well. I was, therefore, assuming the role of a meta-physician—a physician in transformation.

Ultimately, this would all lead me to another level of service—in treating my patients, in teaching my students, and in writing about the concepts that have changed my life in a way that I hope will make an impact on others!

Part II

The Metaphysical Journey

2

Metaphysics—What Does It Mean?

The most beautiful experience we can have is the mysterious. It is the fundamental emotion which stands at the cradle of true art and true science.... A knowledge of the existence of something we cannot penetrate, our perceptions of the profoundest reason and the most radiant beauty.... In this sense, and in this sense alone, I am a deeply religious man.

—Albert Einstein, physicist

A rational explanation for the world in a sense of a closed and complete system of logical truths is almost certainly impossible. We are barred from ultimate knowledge.... We have to embrace a different concept of understanding.... Possibly the mystical path is the way to such an understanding.

—Paul Davies, physicist

Metaphysics. What does it really mean? Allow me to introduce this ancient and often misunderstood term to you. There is no reason to fear it! It is actually quite tame, and sometimes, warm and fuzzy. Much more important, it will help you make sense of your life!

Metaphysics is, literally, the study of the nature of reality. It is the study of what is real and true about the universe, about ourselves, about the nature of God, the afterlife, the soul. It helps us understand whether our lives have any grand purpose, clarifies the nature of "evil," and of suffering.

Metaphysics encompasses the most important questions that any one of us can ask about ourselves and the universe around us. True, it is "officially" a branch of philosophy. Some academics, in fact—those married to metaphysics as an intellectual tradition—will complain that I am using the term too loosely.

Perhaps I am putting my own spin on the topic, but after all, I *am* a physician, and I know many individuals who offer medical advice without a license! An even more fascinating association with metaphysics and my profession is this—how concepts of healing merge with our purpose for being. Kabbalistic notions of *tikkun* or repair/healing are connected with the notion that the universe is fragmented and incomplete—on purpose! Humanity's role becomes that of cocreator with God, of healing that which is incomplete or fragmented. When understood in this grand metaphysical sense, healing becomes the goal of all human existence.

GHOSTS, MEDIUMS, AND MAGIC, OH REALLY?

There are some who will automatically associate metaphysics with the occult, parapsychology, the paranormal, and a vast spectrum of New Age beliefs and activities. This is a strong aspect of the common cultural meaning of the word and it is not *completely* wrong. Some of these can indeed fall under the umbrella of metaphysics.

However, there is much more to metaphysics than these topics alone. My metaphysical umbrella is a big one and there is room enough to fit many different beliefs and approaches to life. To me, *any* form of human expression, exploration, thought, or activity that seeks to extend knowledge, enhance awareness, dispel fear, or explain the unknown becomes metaphysical in nature. For example:

Walking on the beach, listening to the roar of the ocean, feeling the ebb and flow of the water on your feet, and pondering the existence of God is a metaphysical experience.

Offering money to a disheveled beggar is a metaphysical moment. It dissolves boundaries, it shows compassion for another living soul, and it may just move someone from utter despair and potential suicide to a realization that there is kindness in a world preoccupied with self-centered pursuits.

The act of offering compassion to another takes us out of our own self-centered worries and concerns. In the moment of giving, past and future do not exist, and we find ourselves in a sanctuary of peaceful healing.

Learning a new skill, a new fact, a new language, a new concept all contribute to making one more complete, more well-rounded, less ignorant. These are examples of healing and correction as well because they represent a realization of our soul's potential in this world.

Actively pursuing a particular job you want, and discovering you did not get it can cause great disappointment and result in feelings of low self-esteem and sadness. Regarding that disappointment as an opportunity to re-evaluate our strengths and weaknesses with a eye towards learning and growing is a metaphysical experience.

Dealing with an illness makes us feel vulnerable and weak. We feel dependent on those around us, on physicians, on medication. It is a time when we can slip into despair. Yet it is an opportunity to review our personal values. What is truly important to us, friends, family, and loved ones, will remain in our consciousness. The less significant but daily annoyances will vanish like a cloud. To recall this truth when we feel well again is a metaphysical insight.

- Taking a moment to reflect on how our thoughts and feelings produce physical symptoms is a metaphysical moment.
- Caretaking a loved one through a serious health crisis such as cancer, trying to help them live and heal, and ultimately having to watch them die, can be

a heartbreaking experience. However, seeing a loved one's death after such a courageous battle is a lesson on living, dying, and loving—a metaphysical lesson.

Seen in this light—science becomes a form of metaphysics because it is dedicated to uncovering new insights about the nature of the natural world. It seeks to uncover the mystery of existence through a method that requires verification and substantiation of results. It seeks to understand how the universe works. It seeks to dispel ignorance and, through technological advances, improve the quality of life for millions. Less starvation, better medical care, treatment of chronic diseases, and prolongation of meaningful life can be attributed to scientific advances.

Religion seeks to uncover the nature of God, of humankind, and the relationship between the two. In this sense, religion is clearly a metaphysical undertaking as well. It offers institutionalized rituals for dealing with painful transitions, such as death and well-known and comforting practices for birth, marriage, and rites of passage. At its best, religion can incorporate spirituality into the daily lives of individual human beings and helps guide us to a more soulful and thoughtful life.

When viewing metaphysics from this broad spectrum of interpretation, even artistic expression can be regarded as a metaphysical undertaking. Music, art, and literature often reflects the deep desire of the artist to make a statement about what is important in the world, significant in his or her life, and therefore real, if only because they say so, write it, paint it, or create it. Think of it this way:

Music. You can hear a piece of jazz, a song, or an uplifting piece of music and it can vibrate through your body, mind, and soul and uplift you, change your attitude or bring you to a new place of understanding. Perhaps this relates to the universal human activity of creating and listening to music. Repeating mantras, prayers, and chanting have produced characteristic findings on SPECT scans of the brain and been associated with relaxation and feelings of cosmic unity.

And there is art. You can stand for hours gazing at a great work of art hanging on a museum wall and reflect on what the artist is saying. Each moment brings you deeper into the experience of the painting, and each color and brush stroke can tell a story. The position of people, their expressions, objects, nature, forms—considering each is a metaphysical experience.

Think of great books. They are pages and words pressed between two covers, yet a compelling story can transport you to another world where you are on a journey with living, breathing characters. And there are movies and theater experiences that invite you in to try and solve a mystery or understand the motivation of the characters. It can move you, scare you, enlighten you, make you cry, laugh, and focus your mental energy on trying to get the deeper meaning.

Similarly, metaphysics is fluid and changeable. It gives you the opportunity to explore, and even change your mind and select a different point of view or experience. It does not lock you into a mindset, other than "Be open-minded."

Life always gives us choices, and metaphysical awareness is similar to the choice between watching a 3-D movie with or without the special eye gear. Without it, you can still get the gist of the story, but with your 3-D glasses, a much more exuberant and vital set of images emerge. Seeing life through metaphysical eyes gives you the ability to look deeper, appreciate the nuances, study more angles, and explore greater possibilities for healing and wellness.

WHERE *METAPHYSICS* COMES FROM

The word *metaphysics* itself is derived from the body of writing of the Greek philosopher and early scientist Aristotle. It was "discovered," or compiled, by a later scholar, Andronicus of Rhodes. These series of writings, which Aristotle referred to as his "First Philosophy," were uncovered "after his works on the physical world [physica]" The Greek prefix "meta" in this case refers to "after." These writings became known as Aristotle's Metaphysics.

The need to make sense of the world around has been ongoing since the beginning of time and is reflected in the book of Genesis itself.

Adam and Eve risked everything, including immortality, in order to get a taste of the Tree of Knowledge of Good and Evil. Although portrayed by some traditionalists as the origin of Original Sin and the fall of humanity, later Kabbalists interpreted this event to represent the dawn of human consciousness, an event that God *knew* would occur.

Sufis also believe that the story in Genesis is symbolic of the maturation of children having to leaving their father's house in order to explore the world, to learn, and to begin the evolution of humanity. If they had stayed, Adam and Eve would have remained as children or adolescents, unable or incapable of making free will decisions. This rattles those who take the Bible literally because under this scenario, Eve was *meant* to eat the apple. It is a metaphor for the dawning of human consciousness.

A fascinating aspect of the debate on *metaphysics* involves the relationship between philosophy and science. As science grew in stature as a source of truth about the universe, philosophers themselves began to question the validity of *metaphysics* as worthy of study.

Philosophers such as David Hume and Immanuel Kant in the eighteenth and nineteenth century, and Bertrand Russell and A. J. Ayers in the twentieth century declared *metaphysics* to be clearly inferior to science as a source of knowledge.

Intuition, subjective personal experiences, spiritual and paranormal encounters were rejected by philosophers as useless and invalid because they could not be verified by scientific methods.

Ironically, with the introduction of relativity and quantum theory into twentieth-century science, there emerged a paradoxical but fascinating body of metaphysical writing by some of the world's most prestigious physicists. Men such as Albert Einstein, Erwin Schrodinger, Sir Arthur Eddington, Sir James Jeans, John Wheeler, and others were led by their discoveries from science to write about their profound awe at the true nature of reality.

Their work was leading them to make conclusions about the universe that were very clearly mystical in their content. Physicist John Wheeler noted, "There may be no such thing as the glittering central mechanism of the universe.... Not machinery but magic may be the better descriptions of the treasure that is waiting."

Physicist Nick Herbert noted, in discussing mathematician John Von Neuman, "his logic leads to a particularly bizarre conclusion, that by itself the physical world is not fully real, but takes shape only as a result of the acts of numerous centers of consciousness."

EINSTEIN, A META-PHYSICIAN?

> Everyone who is seriously involved in the pursuit of science becomes convinced that a spirit is manifest in the laws of nature—a spirit vastly superior to that of man.

This statement by Einstein was deeply personal and highly controversial. While other scientists may have refused to make metaphysical statements based on their scientific discoveries, Einstein did not. He acknowledged that there are powerful truths that exist beyond the "facts" that science can provide. He acknowledged this basic human need to reach conclusions about the nature of reality.

Other scientists will claim that their research contradicts the existence of a spiritual universe. Finding no evidence for God, they declare that atheism is the only reasonable position to take. They may be unaware that this conclusion is itself metaphysical in nature. It may be just as reasonable to conclude that science cannot "explore" a realm of existence that exists beyond its instruments or methods.

LET'S GET METAPHYSICAL

Our species is clearly compelled to make sense of the world around us as well as the mind within us. This effort can be the source of great comfort as well as confusion and grief. It is important to note, any summation, conclusion, or comment on the ultimate nature of things is *metaphysics*, regardless of its source and content. Awareness of this truth is important.

There are many people who find organized religion provides these kinds of answers for them. For them there are holy books and religious structures that support them in their daily life and guide them through times of darkness.

However, there are many others, who do not find themselves called to a religious path. In fact:

- They find religion to be inadequate to satisfy all their metaphysical needs.
- They are fascinated by ideas, thoughts, and concepts that come from diverse backgrounds, such as science, other spiritual or philosophic traditions.
- They resist religious dogma that tells them they are "sinful" by nature.

- They do not feel that life's difficulties are forms of punishment.
- They may reject the notion that they are victims of life's circumstances.
- They may strongly reject the dogma, tribalistic bias, and intolerance that religions seem to exhibit.

These are individuals I would consider meta-physicians. The hallmark is that they are interested and willing to explore these concepts for themselves. They are skeptical but open-minded. They may actually recognize that life is a training ground for their soul's development.

They are the people who look to the heavens and ask, why? To my mind, meta-physicians are those who embody many of the above qualities, and give themselves permission to question, permission to grow, permission to learn, and permission to heal.

3

Truth about the Metaphysical Journey—Embracing the Power to Choose

> If you would only realize that nothing that comes to you is negative. All trials and tribulations ... are gifts to you. It is an opportunity to grow. This is the whole purpose of existence on this plane.
>
> —Elizabeth Kubler-Ross

The metaphysical journey is never simple or straightforward. Life leads us into seemingly blind cul-de-sacs, endless featureless vistas, and unrecognizable terrain. We often feel lost and confused, without direction or hope. We wonder: Why are we here? Is this the result of random, mindless wanderings? Could there be a purpose to these diversions, these dead ends? Can we actually learn by being lost?

When in a crisis, it can be difficult to believe that we can transform fear into an adventure in learning. When in pain, it may be tough to consider that life's "side excursions" may actually be opportunities for exploration and growth. This, however, is the hallmark of the metaphysical journey—a path with many forks in the road and many unanticipated events.

Perhaps we all need to be more aware of the opportunities that life presents to us every day—and in every moment. The notion that we can actually *choose* what we *want* to believe seems confusing, even nonsensical. Isn't there just one way to understand reality? Wouldn't any other interpretation be just a fantasy or delusion?

Many of us simply are not taught about the true power of the mind. We are not encouraged to write and direct the story of our own lives. So it is understandable that the power to choose, at first, is not a comfortable topic.

CHOOSING HOW WE DEAL WITH CHALLENGE

Many schools of belief tell us that humans come to earth for a reason. Many traditions are based strongly on reincarnation as a very normal part of the cycle of existence. From that perspective, we learn that life's difficulties are necessary for our soul's evolution.

Many spiritual teachings describe the process by which we make agreements or "contracts" prior to our "incarnation" in any particular lifetime. Our souls accepted these challenges, however irrational they may now appear, knowing that by overcoming adversity they could achieve spiritual advancement.

Whether reincarnation seems reasonable to you or not, crisis and challenge has a very practical effect on our growth. "Whatever doesn't kill you ... makes you stronger" is a powerful statement whose source has been attributed to philosopher Friedrich Nietzsche. But this makes sense only if we learn from these predicaments and obstacles. It is balanced by another cliché: "You are only given as much as you can take." These two phrases together alert us to the need to dig down within ourselves, as well as to call upon the assistance of those close to us, to retrieve the resources and strength with which to continue on.

Confusion and chaos in our lives leads to feelings of being out of control. Our minds play and replay our worries and fears about past and future predicaments. This, I believe, is the source of a significant amount of anxiety and depression. The challenge, therefore, is to recognize this truth and to discover mechanisms by which we can assert some element of control within our lives.

Spiritual traditions from both Eastern and Western sources describe the power of living in the moment. It is amazing how difficult this is for us. We are so often bouncing from past to future that the present slips past and evaporates from our lives. The mystical present, the "power of now," is a place of peace and a source of spiritual energy for us. It is accessible through forms of meditation.

This may all seem like a waste of time to us. We must focus on the "real" events in our lives, mustn't we? We seem to be rushing around in all directions, yet often without focus. Stopping and giving ourselves permission to disengage from the chaos around us seems counterproductive. But paradoxically, it is just the opposite.

First, it is crucial to recognize and acknowledge that it is our *minds* that are creating these thoughts and feelings through their filtering and interpretation of events in our lives. Stepping back from the chaos of the mind can be achieved through a variety of techniques: Mindfulness meditation, prayer, forms of yoga, aerobic physical exercise, or other diversions are invaluable. Positive affirmations—telling ourselves that we are capable, loving, and valuable human beings are incredibly powerful tools for healing as well.

CHOOSING THE FILTER THROUGH WHICH WE SEE LIFE

We can choose to view life as a constant challenge to our sense of fairness and peace; something that beats us down. Or we can choose to view it as a cosmic game we are playing. It is a game that *challenges* the belief that we are passive victims of life's difficulties. It gives us power!

Free will is humanity's greatest gift. But this gift brings with it enormous responsibilities: we can choose to accept fear as a necessary consequence of existence. We can accept pain and suffering as a part of the human experience. Or we can become aware that our perspective on fear and pain can either increase or greatly reduce our suffering. We can choose how we view our lives. It is the only power we have in the face of adversity. Nowhere do we see this more powerfully than in our health and well-being.

We may never choose to give up the "struggle." We may not want to *really* overcome our darkest fears—and perhaps we won't. We need, however, to continuously check progress along this chosen path. The weight of despair and discomfort will lift as we see signs of progress, the fruits of our choices. As we see chaos retreating and order and control begin to emerge, we will relax and enjoy the process itself.

4

Solving Life's Mysteries—Why We Search for Knowledge

> The metaphysical quest is man's primary endeavor. The need to comprehend the nature of reality calls upon all our available resources. Science and religion are man's primary tools in this grand undertaking.
>
> —*S. E. Hodes*

Mysteries fascinate human beings. We are drawn to them as if their solution will somehow assist us in our own life's journey. By our very nature, we *love* to solve problems. In fact, we *need* to do so.

It could be that solving life's mysteries actually provides us with the tools we need to control the chaos that surrounds us. And it is precisely this chaos that produces a primal fear—fear of injury, of pain, of loss of our own lives and those of our loved ones. It was this fear that initiated our ancestors' first awareness that they inhabited a dangerous place, filled with uncertainty and pitfalls. It was what led the best and brightest of them to try to understand the mystery, to master *it*—before *it* mastered them.

The mindset of the ancients was not to get smart and become wise. It was to stay alive! It was molded by the hope, and later the belief, that knowledge of the workings of the world would ultimately save them. Their instinctive reasoning went something like this: if the gods were angry, then find out everything you can about these divine beings—their personalities, their likes and dislikes, how to appease them, their favorite sacrifice. Our ancestors learned quickly to do whatever it took—even human sacrifice—to calm the irrational forces that blasted them with life-threatening assaults.

While it may be odd to imagine our forefathers living in the wild and worshipping animals, weather, the sun, the moon, day and night as powerful deities, this is the probable origin of all religions.

Fumbling around in the elements over time and figuring out how the universe operates is most likely the origin of science as well. After all, it seems logical that knowledge of the forces of chaos in the universe might perhaps grant us some sort of control.

THE NATURE OF REALITY

This is exactly where the concept of metaphysics fits in: it is the search for the nature of reality, and it is a search for the key to survival that ultimately and sometimes accidentally evolves into both science and religion.

Understanding the nature of reality is the goal of all metaphysical speculation and it is not for the scholar or mystic alone. There have always been very practical reasons for each of us to explore the universe in which we live. Knowledge of the weather, the seasons, the patterns of animal migrations, the time to plant and harvest crops, the behavior of predatory beasts, the awareness of periods of rain and droughts were all necessary for the survival of our human ancestors.

Knowledge of the unseen universe of spirits and dark forces were necessary for survival as well. Very likely, those who possessed psychic gifts, the shamans, soon rose to prominence as mystical sources of information and power.

Although the world has changed and evolved since the ancients sought to appease the Gods, humans are still seeking ways to unravel the mysteries of life—or at least figure out how to survive in a world that sometimes seems to be spinning out of control.

We seek knowledge (called "gnosis" by the Greeks) in the belief that it will confer some power or influence over the chaos that seems to sometimes overtake our lives. Many of us believe—or secretly dream—it may offer us tools by which to understand, accept, or transform our lives from the day to day confusion that characterizes our daily existence into a more meaningful, joyous experience and appreciation of life.

Some of us continue to try to outrun the "wild animals" and make peace with the gods, but in modern life these become metaphors for the nature and experience of daily living.

Our ancestors took each challenge as a mystery to be solved. Their lives depended on it. We would all benefit from a return to viewing each day as an adventure in living, an opportunity to explore the meaning of existence. Instead of pulling ourselves out of bed each morning with an exasperated sigh, realize that there will never be this particular day, this particular opportunity again. Each day offers unique challenges that at first glance may appear to be another burden for us. There are no useless experiences, only the failure to make the most of them. Wisdom arrives in unexpected packages.

5

Creating Our Own Reality

I believe the mind is the creator of the world and is ever creating.
—Ralph Waldo Emerson

We don't see things as they are, we see them as we are.

—Anaïs Nin

We live in a universe of our own creation. Whether or not we realize this fact, it is true. No other creature sees the world through our eyes, our senses, our brains. Another's perceptions may be more or less intense, more or less colorful, filled with unimagined smells, visions, and sounds. Yet they will never experience the world in the manner in which we do. Even more significant is the fact that no two human beings perceive the exact same world in the exact same way.

An aborigine from the jungles of New Guinea will regard a picture of Jesus or Superman in a far different way than an American in an urban city. Our perceptions occur so rapidly that we fail to realize how edited they are by our memories and emotions. Our brains are unimaginably complex organs, interconnected to our senses. Our belief that our eyes see reality is equally flawed. Every perception of light is filtered through our mind's memory. Emotional content from prior experiences colors everything we experience.

Enter a museum with someone who has a deep love and appreciation of art, a vast knowledge of art history, color, shape, and form. Try to enter their mind as they slowly gather in the shapes and images before them. If you listen to them speak you may be able to absorb a bit of their knowledge and awareness but you will soon realize how much deeper and richer their experience is than your own. You'll find it is literally impossible to "see" what they see.

Clearly, our beliefs about the nature of reality deeply affect how we perceive our own lives. Individuals who see life as difficult, overwhelming, and punishing will find it difficult to find those rare moments of joy and beauty. These persons will likely predict their own suffering, anticipating the next heavy load of pain. They will tend to spread this gloom to all around them.

People who regard life as a joy and a challenge, a source of great opportunity as well as meaningful obstacles to overcome, will undoubtedly experience more balance and peace in their lives. They will, first, seek to find these precious moments. They will shake off defeat as a temporary detour and as a learning experience. They trust in the basic value of themselves as human beings and typically seek the deeper meaning to everything in their lives.

The idea that "things happen for a reason" will be a source of inspiration to them, a source of energy by which to transform disappointment into a new perspective. To pessimists, this idea is more likely to affirm their own status as a victim, someone who is unworthy of happiness or success.

This is not to pretend that life does not present moments of pain and sorrow. That is an aspect of reality we all must acknowledge and accept as inevitable and unavoidable. The suffering and death of those we love, our own physical deterioration and emotional turmoil will often bring a powerful dose of the dark emotions. What separates ultimate healing from ongoing dis*ease* is how we process those feelings. We should not attempt to suppress them. They are a natural and part of life itself. The opportunity is to make peace with grief and despair and understand that they are temporary; although unavoidable they are not impossible to ultimately overcome. Rather than obsess over our worries and troubles, we can learn to allow them to pass through us and trust our own ability to embrace all aspects of living, including the painful aspects.

As much a cliché as it may sound, there is an old adage that fits so well with this line of thinking: "The pessimist sees the glass half empty and the optimist sees the glass half full."

People who tend to see the glass half full often suffer from the belief that their cup will never be full and their thirst will never quite be quenched. I would challenge those folks to at least attempt to flip their perspective and see how life feels when it seems fuller and more balanced.

6

Anatomy of a Belief

No logical path exists between the theoretical concepts and our observations. One is brought into concordance with the other by an "extralogical" or intuitive process.

—Albert Einstein

You are what you believe. Any self-proclaimed meta-physician will readily admit that as a consequence of their journey, they have accumulated a series of beliefs that form the basis for their own metaphysical journey. We often forget to explore exactly *how* we come to embrace these beliefs. It is often as important as what we actually believe to be true.

We need to understand that the process of belief is not simple. It is an amalgam of what we are taught, what we observe, and what we think about all of this, and, perhaps most important, it has an intuitive component as well.

The approach that scientists take regarding their base of knowledge is worth remembering: be willing to reevaluate and reassess all your preconceptions. Nevertheless, there are still many scientists, as well as ordinary human beings, who will often proclaim an open-mindedness while in reality they retreat to the beliefs that they regard as fundamental and unchanging.

In order to truly grow, and heal, we must be open-minded skeptics. Exploring how a belief system comes into being is a tool to creating new, healing choices. It helps us see the connection between mind, body, and spirit.

WHO'S AFRAID OF EPISTEMOLOGY?

In the language of philosophy we are breaking down the concept of *metaphysics* into two component parts: *ontology*, which is the substance of what we believe to be true about the nature of reality, and *epistemology*, the study of knowledge and how we obtain it.

We often forget the sources of our own beliefs but it is important to analyze them a bit. It may be useful to consider the four R's.

Receiving Is Not Always a Gift

The first R is what we "receive." This is an extremely influential and powerful source of our beliefs. It represents the influences we receive from a multitude of sources: teachers, religious leaders, political leaders, the educational system, religious institutions and dogma, mass media, friends, books, and so on. It is important to realize that what we receive (particularly when we are young and impressionable or emotionally vulnerable and unaccustomed to questioning authority) may appear to us to be valid and true. But there is a caveat here—it can lead us into acts that are ultimately destructive and self-destructive.

For example, some of us may grow up in families that have their own biased beliefs about other racial, religious, or political groups. This perspective will become so ingrained within us that it may be quite difficult to view these positions from any other point of view.

Often, the source of stereotyping other groups of people arises from a fear of the other. The response to this fear is either to withdraw completely or, conversely, to aggressively seek to destroy that which is feared. Either response is self-defeating and can lead to a vicious cycle of further insecurity and fear.

The same dynamics occur within any individuals who may be raised with personal biases that promote a negative attitude toward people of different backgrounds. It may keep them in a state of reactive fear, unable to express openness and to perceive and receive the beauty and kindness inherent in others.

It is particularly disheartening to realize how children can be inculcated with hatred towards others of divergent religious or racial background. Such deeply ingrained lessons are extremely difficult to alter. This, to my mind, is unquestionably a form of metaphysical child abuse, one that has horrendous global implications for war and peace.

Blind Faith Takes a Leap

Issues of belief involve those of faith versus evidence. This becomes somewhat controversial since some religious doctrines promote the leap of faith and a rejection of rational thought or experience. "Just believe," "Keep the faith," and "Trust in the Lord" form the basis of many belief systems of individuals. This metaphysical perspective certainly makes changing one's mind or reconsidering a belief rather unlikely.

There are others, like myself, who are not persuaded by exhortations to have faith. We need evidence. Even if we cannot explain all the metaphysical implications of this evidence, we are somewhat more empirical in our demands. We tend to be more scientific in that we are open to new evidence and new analysis of the information we receive.

In his book *The Universe in a Single Atom*, the Dalai Lama, spiritual leader of Tibetan Buddhists, acknowledges that what we believe must be evidence-based. He even states that if science proves a concept that is contrary to Buddhist scripture, the scripture, and not science, must change. He finds no conflict between science and spirituality. Science studies the physical world, and spirituality comprehends morality and meaning.

What we receive also involves what our senses tell us about the natural world. Most neuroscientists and many philosophers have demonstrated either by science or logic that our perceptions are filtered through the doors of our own minds and, therefore, are not reliable indicators of ultimate reality. It is one reason, I regret, that some seekers have abandoned the search for truth.

Philosopher Immanuel Kant has been credited with bringing the notion of metaphysics to its knees by noting that we can never truly *know* what is ultimately real because of the filtering of the human mind. Quantum theory has supported this notion that the nature of an experiment—how it is observed—affects the actual outcome. Light can be determined to be either a particle or a wave, all depending on the experimental setup.

But knowing the nature of the human mind will not diminish our desire to seek ultimate metaphysical truth.

There are powerful neural connections between our optic input and the emotional and memory centers of our brain. There is little question that a Holocaust survivor will see a picture of Hitler in a much different way than an aboriginal inhabitant of the Brazilian rain forest. Likewise, the sight of a particular bird or lizard will evoke a much different response in the Brazilian than in someone raised in a major urban city.

Limitations of Reason

"Reason" is another R that deserves consideration. Traditionally, philosophers known as rationalists have argued that reason alone can bring us ultimate metaphysical awareness. Plato wrote about the Ideal Forms that exist apart from the world of our senses. Proof of God's existence were metaphysical exercises that were more about how we defined God as the ultimate creator, designer, or being, rather than any real "proof."

Science and spirituality are not inherently contradictory metaphysical perspectives. The use of reason may, however, be seen by organized religion as rather threatening. It may challenge the validity of any one religion in view of the large numbers that exist.

After all, there is one physics, one chemistry, and one biology that apply to all of humanity. Similarly, the great spiritual traditions of antiquity have always sought unification with the Creator or Absolute Spirit. Reason would suggest, therefore, that the multiplicity of religions represent historical and cultural differences that have evolved into separate organizations whose main objective is not truth but self-preservation. This, however, does not automatically reject the deeper mystical heart that all religions claim is their spiritual core. Especially in the face of what should be one metaphysical truth to all.

Science and reason can surely embrace with sensitivity and humility the great mystery of existence. In fact, contemporary science is clearly demonstrating that the deeper it peers into the abyss, the deeper the darkness. In fact, the concepts of dark energy and dark matter only add to the awe and mystery of existence.

This drive to find a unified explanation for reality seems to be a basic human desire. Although ultimately incorrect, the early Greek philosopher/scientists each picked a different primary substance—water, fire, air, or water—to be seen as the basis of reality.

The attempt to reconcile conflicting fields of Relativity Theory and Quantum Mechanics was an unrealized attempt by Einstein to find the Theory of Everything. To him this was a spiritual goal: to ultimately believe that intuition was needed to bridge the gap between reason and the experience of science.

Be Reasonable?

The danger is, reason can lead us through logic to erroneous beliefs. That is because if we begin with an incorrect premise, our ability to use logic and reason will lead only to incorrect conclusions. A fundamental belief that certain religions or races of people are inherently inferior led to logically derived laws and assumptions that have had horrific consequences.

At the conclusion of the nineteenth century, science students were being dissuaded from studying physics because the assumption was that only "two small clouds" of ignorance persisted in the Newtonian mechanistic view of the universe. Ultimately, these two small clouds led to Relativity and the Quantum Theory. This is why Einstein also insisted that the concepts of reason be checked against the findings of experience, and why he embraced intuition or revelation as a source of potential wisdom.

Question Everything

We will tend to incorporate those beliefs and opinions, seeing them as true without questioning their basic assumptions. The ability of groups to commit genocide, war, and dehumanization of other groups demonstrates the power of "group think" to see ourselves as isolated, defensive tribal units. The often extolled golden rule of "do unto others as you would them do unto you" is denied when we are brainwashed to see our fellow human beings as inferior, or to simply see ourselves as more entitled than others.

This is one of the most powerful reasons individuals should always assert their individual freedom to question and to challenge authority regarding that which is contrary to what seems right. Failure to do so has led to the most despicable of human behavior.

From a spiritual perspective, we each carry our individual deeds with us from one lifetime to another. This is the true meaning of karma. We are not absolved because we were only "following orders," nor, I believe, by merely having faith in the redemptive power of another being.

From a perspective of healing, we should not automatically believe that physicians can predict our medical futures. We can choose to "give up" hope or to pursue reasonable alternatives. There is a world of what is known as complementary and alternative medicine [CAM] and writers such as Kenneth R. Pelletier, Ph.D., Daniel J. Benor, M.D., Jane E. Brody, and Denise Grady and others have researched what actually works. They explore acupuncture, homeopathy, naturopathy, herbal therapy, energy modalities, and a host of treatments and philosophies that diverge from traditional medical practices.

We may not be aware of the power of the mind to facilitate healing, to empower our immune system, to soothe our suffering. We must constantly monitor those free choices and evaluate the risk versus the benefit of any of these decisions.

Who Turned on the Light?

Another R is "revelation." Similar to concepts of intuition and insight, this is a particularly complex subject and not as easy to define. It is not science and it cannot be replicated under experimental conditions. It is the essence of mystical insights that form the basis of all established religions. These episodes may arise spontaneously or as a result of practiced methods of meditation, prayer, and contemplation. Unfortunately, religions can become petrified, dogmatic institutions that discourage new examples of revelation. It is as though they accept the revelations of the past, which they have frozen into their doctrines and canon of writings and assume that mankind is no longer spiritually connected.

William James, M.D., studied these mystical experiences in the later nineteenth and early twentieth century. His American Society of Psychical Research promoted a rational, evidence-based, and scientific examination of the claims of mystics and mediums, and his *Varieties of Religious Experiences* is a landmark work in the entire field.

Psychologist Lawrence LeShan has likewise applied rational approaches with an open-minded skepticism to these subjects and has concluded that there is much evidence to justify a belief in their veracity.

A host of researchers, such as Raymond Moody, M.D., Ph.D., Kenneth Ring, Ph.D., Peter Fenwick, M.D., and Elisabeth Kubler-Ross, M.D., have openly and rationally studied the near-death experience and concluded that, rather than a hallucinatory delusion associated with hypoxia (lack of oxygen to the brain), it seems to reveal a mystical reality.

But revelation is not dead. Individuals seem to have mystical experiences at all times in all cultures under a variety of circumstances. They may be termed paranormal or spiritual: Near-death experiences, out-of-body experiences, clairvoyant perceptions, after-death communication, and a host of other unexplained experiences seem to describe another level of reality that cannot be reached by what is received from others or via reason.

Psychologist Gary Schwartz has systematically studied the abilities of contemporary mediums to provide information regarding deceased loved ones. His conclusions, including the use of controlled studies, have been extremely favorable toward the truth of the mediums' experiences.

The presence of spiritual or paranormal experiences among ordinary, sane human beings cannot be ignored. I have been fortunate enough to have been entrusted with these deeply personal and emotional encounters with another level of reality.

Ranging from near-death experiences, to after-death communications, to experiences with psychics and mediums, they have become the fuel for my journey to understand the nature of reality.

Feel the Beat

The final R is "resonance." It is the sum total of the experiences, perceptions, thoughts, feelings, and beliefs that constitute what we believe to be true. It incorporates what we receive from those around us, including our senses, what our minds logically tell us is true, and perhaps, if we are fortunate, some mystical insights.

It is the ultimate basis for what we all believe to be true. It encompasses all other inputs—what we receive, what our reason tells us, and even our spiritual revelations. It is the present state of our metaphysical belief. But it should never be set in stone. This does not mean that the ultimate truth changes. It only implies that our awareness evolves.

How can we actively evolve our awareness and adapt our beliefs? Continue to read and study. Continue to gaze at the wonder of nature, of new life, even of the intensity and reality of death. Immerse yourself in deep thought, meditation, contemplation, and prayer. "Try on" different beliefs. See what fits best. Your inner knowing will resonate with what is right for you.

Open yourself up to an increased awareness of the mystery that surrounds you. It may be that we are constantly offered gifts of joy and insight but we just don't slow down or relax enough to perceive them. Nurture your beliefs. They will guide you. They are the paradigm through which you create your own reality.

Part III
Science and Mind

We have found that where science has progressed the farthest, the mind has but regained from nature that which the mind has put into nature.... We have found a strange footprint on the shores of the unknown.... At last, we have succeeded in reconstructing the creature that made the footprint. And lo! It is our own.

—Arthur Eddington, physicist

7

Healing the Heart–Mind Divide

We think by feeling, what is there to know?

—Theodore Roethke, poet

Thinking versus feeling. Objective versus subjective. Science versus spirituality.

Are these irreconcilable opposites? Can we ever hope to bring a deeper understanding to what would appear to be such different perspectives on the nature of reality?

We often hear the expression "be reasonable" or "use your head, not your heart" in discussing issues of public or personal concern. The same difficulties that individuals deal with in their daily lives, in their interpersonal relationships, seem to occur between nations as well. Perhaps that is because thinking and feeling are so intimately connected that attempting to separate them is virtually pointless.

Science has clearly demonstrated its phenomenal ability to better the lives of the vast majority of human beings on this planet. Technological advancements in medical care, communications, food production, and exploration of the cosmos cannot be denied. But are individuals any happier than they were a century ago? Although their brains may be filled with sophisticated concepts and more knowledge, are their hearts any more content, at ease?

The truth is: we may try to be rational, logical beings; we may struggle to educate ourselves, be open-minded regarding a variety of issues, and be tolerant and reasonable, but we live in our hearts. It is extremely difficult to alter or undo our childhood influences regarding racial and religious bigotry—precisely because these feelings are so deeply entrenched.

The all-too-frequent spontaneous racial or ethnic slurs by celebrities and public figures, who should "know better," are far from rare. These have been, at times, blamed on excessive drug or alcohol consumption. But true feelings are often revealed in such moments of unguarded candor.

The present indoctrination of children around the world into fundamentalist beliefs that demean or indict other human beings is particularly dangerous and damaging. Such ingrained beliefs carry powerful emotional anchors.

But history clearly shows that religion is not the sole culprit in such abominable activities. Two of the twentieth century's most horrific movements were antireligious. Hitler's Germany and Stalin's Soviet Empire perpetrated slaughter and genocide on the basis of fundamentalist beliefs that tapped into humanity's most vulnerable emotion—fear.

The distinction between objective and subjective reality is equally questionable. Mystics and philosophers alike acknowledge that all reality is filtered through the prism of our own minds or consciousness. Even quantum physicists have acknowledged that we cannot eliminate the influence of our own testing of the physical world on what actually exists. Terms such as "observer influence" and "the problem of measurement" are troubling concepts to physicists because they indicate that the act of measuring a quantum experiment in which photons or electrons may exist as either a wave or particle produces one or the other—but not both—results. This complex and confusing concept (even to quantum physicists) suggests to some that there is no way to comprehend a world distinct from human consciousness.

Certainly there is something out there, the basis for our perceptions of the external world. But what that is, apart from our interpretation, is totally unclear. In effect, we all do create our own reality. When we communicate well with others, our individual subjective realities seem to coincide with each other. We seem to touch an inner core of our shared humanity that transcends mere words. Empathy and compassion between two individuals are often communicated by nonverbal means—a glance, a sigh, a touch, a tear. These are more powerful than any spoken words.

The dynamic tension between our innate ability to think and to feel might well be the source of great art—literature, music, theater, and painting. But while these two powerful aspects of human consciousness may be the source of great love poems, they can also lead to confusion and chaos.

The artistic temperament is often associated with such intense expressions of feelings and the irrepressible desire to express them. Yet few societies do not honor the unique artists within their ranks. We observe the personal eccentricities of actors, rock stars, artists. We seem to understand that a bit of madness comes with the territory. However, we may be less willing to tolerate such behavior from our accountant, attorney, or physician. These are professionals whose guidance we seek because of their ability to use their cognitive powers with precision, reason, and logic.

Our visual perceptions, seemingly free of emotional aspects, are, in fact, the result of inputs from our memories and the emotional center of our brains An image of Jesus will evoke much different thoughts and feelings from members of a Pentecostal church than a group of committed atheists. The distinction between thinking and feeling often becomes blurred. We may frequently deceive ourselves in our belief that we can be objective about politics, religion, and our personal relations.

Our personal experiences, emotional histories, and individual temperaments influence how we view the world around us. Have you ever met a person who in some way reminded you of someone you either like or dislike intensely? Of course, this happens to all of us. Recall how we viewed that individual, how we judged him or her often before he or she said even one word! Yet we may very well judge ourselves as fair, open-minded, and rational human beings.

GOING INWARD

Many spiritual traditions recognize the necessity to train the mind to rein in the chaotic excesses of the head's monkey-chatter of thoughts and the heart's cascade of emotions. Only when we feel a sense of some control over how we think and feel can we find some sense of peace within our lives.

Mystics of all spiritual traditions have found the discipline of prayer, meditation, and contemplation to be a vehicle by which one's mind or consciousness can exert some influence on the wild—and often debilitating—gyrations of the heart and emotions.

Going *inward* can be a way to heal the heart–mind divide. It becomes a way of gaining access to divine guidance and compassion. It means stepping out of the flow of time, stopping the rush of activities and thoughts that overwhelm us. It means being present in the moment: through meditation, or prayer, or gazing at a leaf on a tree or at an ant scurrying along the ground. Going inward allows one to find peace in the midst of chaos. It helps discipline the mind, and therefore the emotions.

For going inward to achieve a greater meaning, we must take what we receive and learn, and share its wisdom with others who may still be suffering. It can become a lesson in healing for all involved.

8

Science and Spirituality: Metaphysics of the Unexplained

I maintain that the cosmic religious feeling is the strongest and noblest motive for scientific research.

—Albert Einstein

Science has earned its reputation as the source of incredible knowledge about the physical universe. Its methods have evolved over several centuries of debate and discussion. The scientific method involves such a powerful source of knowledge about the world because at its very core is the acknowledgement that scientific knowledge may be temporary and replaceable. Science is always open to be refuted, altered, changed, and enlightened by new experiments and data.

Science searches, it makes observations, it creates hypothesis, it designs experiments, and it publishes the results and opens itself to the review and criticism of others. It evolves publicly, through peer review and discussion with other scientists. Spirituality and religion (organized and institutionalized spirituality), on the other hand, remained personal or communal and always subjective. It could not claim to be provable or demonstrable by objective examination.

For centuries, science seemed to offer all the answers to our questions of existence. Its success, however, brought with it an overconfidence and sense of supremacy over all other paths to knowledge. Before long, some scientists declared that if science cannot study, explain, and prove a phenomenon, it does not exist!

When it came to discussions of the mind, emotions, or feelings, science refused to consider them "real." They were seen as illusions of the mechanistic brain. Anything other than scientifically proven evidence was seen as a delusion or wishful thinking.

Can science truly satisfy any of us, in the long run, as a way of explaining all of life? You may love your kids, your mate, your wide-screen TV, football on Sunday and dancing on Saturday, but do you need to prove it in a laboratory?

Of course not! But if some scientists had their way, we would have those aspects of our consciousness that we cherish most declared irrelevant and less than real.

As humans around the world tap into the deeper, less documented aspect of our existence, science marches on, relegating the study of spirituality and religion to the back burner. Even though some of the hottest books are those with spiritual and metaphysical themes and all media portray a deep interest in the world beyond science, science is, for the most part, preoccupied with itself.

Metaphysical topics such as life after death, after-death communication, the soul, reincarnation, psychic ability, apparitions, and medium encounters are dismissed as pseudo-science.

Still, denying spirituality, God, the soul, life after death, and reincarnation does not mean they do not exist. There is a metaphysical concept that has been ascribed to various spiritual leaders which states that the absence of finding something does not mean it does not exist. Quite simply, you did not find it, that's all. The failure of science to explain the unexplained concepts of spirituality is not evidence of their nonexistence.

My own investigations have led me to believe that these experiences *are real*, they do occur. I have met many individuals who have confided their experiences to me. Many were reluctant to do so, fearing I would find them strange or weird. These honest testimonies have become my evidence for a spiritual reality that I characterize as "the unexplained."

Perhaps these have natural causes. Perhaps they are merely hallucinations, but perhaps they are of a distinctly supernatural nature. At present I prefer to call them unexplained. And I know that they occur to ordinary, sane, and completely credible human beings on a frequent basis. Someday they may be understood to represent a totally different realm of knowledge, or perhaps an as-yet-unknown field of science. Just because science cannot explain them does not make them unreal. To paraphrase a popular notion, "absence of proof is not proof of absence."

Even science cannot completely explain itself. There are a growing number of scientific concepts that can be classified as unexplained. This is in striking contrast to the view science held nearly one hundred years ago. Before the onset of quantum and relativity theory, physicists believed that they had explained the workings of the universe. It was a giant machine, with all its various parts and mechanisms available to the mind of humanity.

How is it possible that in the beginning of the twenty-first century, there is so much in science that is unexplained? In his book *The End of Science*, John Horgan explores several of these remaining mysteries, including the fact that scientists still:

- Do not understand what came before the Big Bang.
- Do not understand how the mind works.
- Cannot explain the origin of life.
- Cannot explain how autistic savants can perform incredible mathematical or musical feats with the IQ of someone who is retarded.
- Cannot explain why they only recently came to realize that all the matter that they can see and measure in the universe only represents about 4 percent of the total. (The rest is dark energy and dark matter).
- Cannot measure the momentum and location of an object at the same time without disrupting the measurement of the other.

- Cannot bring relativity theory and quantum theory together into a coherent theory of everything.

This is terribly disturbing to science. Scientists believed that they had the only key to unlocking the mysteries of the universe. But it seems as if the lock has been changed. The more they peer through their instruments, check their equations, scratch their heads, the less certain they are that they know what is going on.

Rather than throw out what science cannot study, perhaps we better take a closer look at it. Perhaps the unexplained is leading us along a path toward something more profound than science alone can take us.

9

Are We Ever Out of Our Minds?

I believe the mind is the creator of the world and is ever creating.
—Ralph Waldo Emerson

The greatest discovery of my generation is that a human being can alter his life by altering his attitudes of mind.
—William James

What is the mind? We tend to think of it as the "brain," and as something that resides within the confines of our "heads." In everyday life it would seem to be home for our thoughts and feelings as well as the internal battleground upon which the events of our daily lives play themselves out. We seem to jump from event to event, thought to thought, and feeling to feeling, often without any sense of coherence or direction.

It might seem that we tend to cling to familiar thoughts and images. And the mind seems to direct us to habitual ways of living, eating, and thinking. Essentially untrained, uninhibited, and out of control, our minds seems to take us on a fast-moving train ride each day. This chaos is, in itself, a source of anxiety. The harder we try to exert our will, the more illusive is the coherence and balance.

Is the mind one and the same as the brain? Is it the powerful synthesizer of reality or an illusion, merely the "emergent" product of the electrochemical transmissions of the brain? Neurophysiologists and mystics might agree to disagree. *Emergent* is used to describe how something as incredible as the mind, or consciousness, can form as a result of neural and electrochemical processes. Essentially it is a descriptive term that doesn't explain how this actually happens. To say that the mind emerges is to say we really have no clue how we are conscious beings with thoughts. But at least we have a word that describes the mystery of the mind.

Here's some food for thought: What if the brain doesn't produce the mind at all? What if the individual mind—yours and mine—reflect, or is, an inherent property of the universe? What if the brain is simply a transmitter of the mind or consciousness, in the way a radio tunes into signals that would otherwise be undetected and unknown. Philosopher David Chalmers believes the mind is a fundamental force in the universe, like gravity, which is not derived from anything else. It just *is*.

In our usual state of consciousness, we humans believe ourselves to actually be our thoughts and emotions. We find it difficult, if not absurd, to comprehend any other state of awareness. Meditation may be the solution to the contemporary dis*ease* of the chaotic mind. As old as human consciousness, it is a haven of peace in a sea of trouble. Although there are many forms of meditation, it seems to me that mindfulness is a practical and useful approach toward healing the "monkey chatter" of our minds. In this meditative exercise, we observe our thoughts and feelings. We are the witness—we do not try to ignore or suppress them. We observe them as one would a series of floating clouds.

The metaphysical implications are profound.

This method centers on an awareness and focus on the in-and-out flow of the breath. Ideas and feelings that are the residue of the restless mind are allowed to float into consciousness and then to leave the same way. When we become aware that we have been entertaining a thought or emotion, we can then redirect our awareness to the breath. All this is done with a sense of peace and calm. When we slip back into the flow of thoughts, we can catch ourselves and, with infinite patience, calmly redirect our attention back to the breath. Practice improves the performance and the state of calm that ensues.

If we are not our thoughts or emotions—then who are we? Buddhists would insist that our Higher Self—our higher consciousness—is what we are.

Is the mind the same as the soul? There is great controversy over this point as well. The mind may be the soul's manifestation, in the physical form. The mind may be that aspect of the soul which creates and reacts in any one lifetime. No matter. The mind is our "home" in any one lifetime. We had better organize the clutter if we are to escape the chaos that surrounds us.

10

Are We Hard-Wired for Bliss?

Too much of a good thing can be wonderful!

—Mae West

It is clear to me that we *Homo sapiens* evolved with the innate physical and chemical structure to be happy. Let me explain: According to Darwinian theory, those of our ancestors who were able to find meaning and purpose in life must have had a survival advantage over the more depressed of the tribe. With the onset of human awareness our early ancestors also came to realize that everyone they loved and cared for would die—themselves included. They also acquired the ability to worry about everything. To constantly fear the unknown can clearly produce paralysis and might even lead to suicide. It would seem that a good outlook on life would go a long way toward helping to ensure survival.

Early man needed to balance both the ability to predict possible misfortune and calamity with the ability to move past distress and suffering. Both qualities are clearly manifest in contemporary human behavior and perhaps it is the excess of one over the other that determines the nature and color of individual personalities. Recent studies of human emotions under positron emission tomography (PET) scans have shown that characteristic areas of brain activity light up when someone feels contentment and bliss. Similar effects can be produced by individuals trained in the techniques of meditation.

Critics of the special significance of spiritual experiences will point out that they are merely in the brain and, therefore, not at all mystical or spiritually significant. They would say these are simply electrochemical reactions and not "real."

Of course the response is quite simple—everything is in the brain! Everything we do, say, taste, and experience has a correlate on these scans. Eating an apple, drinking lemonade, having sex—all will be revealed on our PET scans. But no one would question the reality of a sensuous encounter with lemonade, apple pie and a delightful partner. Would they?

That is similar to taking a picture of an elephant, and then looking at the picture and stating, "That is not the elephant." Of course it isn't. It is a representation of a real event, a thing, an object.

We live in a drug culture that insists on prescription and herbal chemicals to improve our moods and attitudes. The fact that these drugs actually work on our brains is proof positive of one thing—our brains have evolved with receptor sites to allow us to feel better, to be less anxious, less depressed, more positive, and joyous. The field of psychoneuroimmunology has clearly provided scientific evidence to ensure us that peace of mind and contentment is associated with higher functioning of our immune system. Therefore, happier means healthier. And since these receptor sites in our brains evolved long before the discovery of drugs, we must all be endowed with the capacity to heal ourselves!

There must be an extraordinary evolutionary reason why our bodies have evolved such structures. Our ancestors who possessed these receptors must have had survival advantages over their contemporaries who did not. That is pure evolutionary theory at play here and it actually makes sense. Those who could calm themselves and maintain functionality in the midst of chaos, were more likely to mate and produce offspring, thereby sending us their receptor genes.

It is extremely important for our fellow humans to understand that we are capable of altering our states of feeling, of consciousness—of finding bliss—and often without the use of external, synthetic compounds that merely mimic our internal peptides. Exercise, meditation, cognitive therapy, prayer, and sex—these are all natural means of realizing our potential to be happy.

This is not to diminish the utility of drugs for specific people under specific circumstances. It is just that we usually seek the quick and simple solution of popping a pill before doing the hard work of seeking alternative solutions. But regardless, it does seem as if God/Universe wants us to experience heaven on earth.

The metaphysical implications are fascinating: We need not feel guilty for seeking pleasure. It is in our nature!

Those of us with spiritual leanings should regard this arrangement as a gift from God. This is a rather prominent perspective of the ancient earth religions as well as from the Kabbalistic perspective. One Hasidic tale speaks of a man who dies and meets God (Jews don't meet Saint Peter). It turned out that during his life the man was plagued by feelings of guilt over his desires to embrace his physical nature: food, drink, sex. He prided himself in his vigilance and ability to live a nearly ascetic life. When he approached God he was rather proud of these efforts. He proudly proclaimed how he struggled to be "good." Rather disappointed, God replied, "That is a shame. Why didn't you partake of these pleasures that I provided for you? After all, you are my taste buds in the world."

The point of the story is to portray the Universe/God as offering us gifts of joy in the face of the obvious existence pain and suffering. The point is to spiritualize them. They are not the Devil's tool to lead us into sin or damnation—unless we *choose* to regard them as such.

The nature of bliss and joy can become an enormously powerful lesson for us. They, too, are spiritual gifts. They challenge us to appreciate and use them in the right way. By this I mean appreciate them, be grateful to them, thank God for them and use them wisely and in a way that is fulfilling.

Can they be perverted? Clearly they can and often are. The Universe tells us that we need to always seek a balance between forces. Sex can be an offering of love or a weapon of violence and degradation. Our taste for food and drink can be balanced, nuanced, and appreciated or can become the object of obsession and damage our health as well as our self-image.

So being hard-wired for bliss is just one aspect of the human experience. It is a part of our lives, offered, I believe, as a counterbalance to the pain and suffering. Like Yin and Yang it is necessary gift. How we choose to use it in our lives is up to us.

11

Darkness and Light

And God said, Let there be Light and there was Light

—Genesis 1:3

And God saw the Light, and said that it was Good and God divided the Light from the Darkness.

—Genesis 1:4

The concept of darkness and light has always had profound metaphysical implications. Light implies a beneficent divine presence, or wisdom. Light has always been associated with the good, or holiness, while dark implies just the opposite.

Kabbalistic texts speak of the Creation as the emanation of light (*Or* in Hebrew) from *Ein Sof* (the unknowable essence of Divinity) into the cosmic vacuum. But as someone drawn into exploring the mystery of existence, I am always open to the paradox that darkness may be as important as light.

Our physical beings, as well, are drawn to light. The nature of living things is that they, by definition, defy the laws of thermodynamics. If the universe had its way, our atoms would be scattered across a billion light-years of space. Instead, we are held together and encased in skin, a mass of living flesh we call "a body."

Life exists because it *insists* on existing. It exists in defiance of the laws of physics, but has managed to do so by grabbing the energy of the stars and drawing it down to serve its purpose. Does this sound like there is some sort of intelligence acting in the nature of life itself? No one can prove that assertion. Yet no one can disprove it either!

IS IT A MIRACLE?

Photosynthesis is the scientific term for a true miracle. Forget about the Shroud of Turin, bleeding stigmata, crying statues, or parting Red Seas. Just ponder what truly happens when a tiny organelle—the chloroplast within the cells of the leaves of green plants grabs on to invisible carbon dioxide gas—soaks up water through its stems and mixes light energy from the sun. It then builds these invisible carbon atoms into its own skeleton, into sugars, into the food that allows animals to live. No animal can do this. No animal can extract the energy of life from a star 93 million miles away. Is this not alchemy at its finest?

What is even more bizarre is the truth that the chloroplasts, the tiny structures that live within the cytoplasm of plant cells, has a DNA structure that differs from the plant's own nuclear DNA. The scientific implications for this are astounding. It signals that a billion years in the past, chloroplasts were free-living bacteria capable of photosynthesis. They were in a joint venture with early plant cells. They stayed and became the machinery of life on this planet.

But most life on this planet derives its energy from the Sun. Science has uncovered some incredible sources of life, far away from sunlight. Known as extremophiles, extremely primitive bacteria as well as larger, plant-like structures have been identified thousands of feet below the ocean's surface, living off the energy derived from volcanic activity at temperatures that would annihilate usual forms of life. These bacterial forms have acquired the capacity to utilize sulfur as well. Some forms can live in extremely high acid, or alkali environments.

So, voila! Life can arise from darkness as well. The womb of their origin is far from the light of the sun. There is a big question mark about the role of light in the overall structure of the universe. Astrophysicists have concluded that everything we see through visible light, as well as every bit of energy detected along the electromagnetic spectrum, represents only 4 percent of reality!

And God said, "Let there be light." So even though light came into being, the darkness remained as something real, yet mysterious. Some scientists propose that dark matter (called dark because it emits no energy at all as we know it) represents 22 percent of the universe and dark energy represents a whopping 74 percent of the rest!

The metaphysical implications of these findings are not even being discussed in scientific circles. Here in the early years of the twenty-first century, science is uncovering a level of reality that they cannot explain. This makes the perplexing topics of relativity and quantum theory look easy. Science may be stumped.

Yet the mystery is appealing as well. Does this open up the possibility of other universes, dimensions of existence, a spiritual dimension to reality? It would not be intellectually honest to jump on all this mystery and proclaim that everything is possible. We need to remain skeptical of such leaps of faith. But by the same token, we should not be slamming the door on the possibility of the unexplained leading us to new metaphysical insights.

Let's not be so quick to deny the possibility of a whole host of paranormal phenomena. "A rational explanation for the world in the sense of a closed and complete system of logical truths is almost certainly impossible," noted physicist Paul Davies. "We are barred from ultimate knowledge. . . . We have to embrace a different concept of understanding. . . . Possibly the mystical path is the way to such an understanding."

DARKNESS AS LIGHT

There is something very special about the darkness that enters our lives. It always appears to us at first as painful, unpleasant, something to run and hide from. Yet it is a part of our lives, a part of everyone's life. No one is immune from negativity, from suffering. It has kept the pens of poets busy over time and is the source of many a book, song, opera, movie and work of art. Theodore Roethke wrote, "In a dark time, the eye begins to see." St. John of the Cross called the spiritual crisis that needed to evolve and mature us "dark night of the soul."

Many see darkness as punishment. In actuality, it is a challenge meant to be overcome and mastered. Many of us who have come through dark times look back upon the experience as painful but transformative.

On this metaphysical quest we must be open to explore all possibilities. Darkness may not be the absence of light but the ultimate womb of creation.

Part IV

Testing Credibility—How Do You Know What's Real?

Thus, from personal experience, as well as from the professional literature in this field, I could no longer doubt the existence of telepathy, clairvoyance, and other paranormal phenomena.

—Lawrence LeShan, Ph.D.

12

The Credibility Quotient

How can I believe you when I often doubt myself?

—S. E. Hodes

What is the nature of reality? This is the primary metaphysical question. Of course, it is a "loaded" question because no one can totally and completely supply the ultimate answer to the satisfaction of everyone. Yet that does not deter us from pursuing the ultimate goal—to understand what is real and know how the universe truly works, so that we can gain some sense of control over the fear and chaos that surrounds us.

We are members of a society and culture that separates religious belief from common sense, as well as empirical and scientific thinking. Many will acknowledge a spiritual reality, but only as it is directed and promoted by organized religion. The personal paranormal and spiritual experiences of others is often rejected as irrational or hallucinatory, or as the work of the devil. It is as if spirituality must be confined to prescribed patterns and religious institutions in order to be real.

However, I find that our understanding of the paranormal and spiritual aspects of metaphysics is an essential element in awakening us to a larger reality—that we are far more than this physical body in which we reside. Without this awareness, we cannot truly understand the meaning of *to heal, to make whole*. We must come to an understanding that "spirit" is real before we can incorporate this into our notion of healing. Without this understanding, we cannot appreciate that true health involves a balanced integration of our body, along with mind and spirit.

For some individuals, organized religion provides this spiritual knowledge and connects to all that is. However, for many others, religion does not resonate with such meaning. Perhaps in the mind of some it is the legacy of religious intolerance that taints its spiritual message. Perhaps it is the narrow interpretation of spirituality along historical and specific, rigid pathways that discourages the acceptance of its deeper spiritual message.

Whatever the reason, there are individuals—like myself—who are open-minded skeptics and obliged by our very nature to do our own metaphysical exploration. There are individuals, like myself, who need evidence for a spiritual dimension to reality—one that involves personal research and exploration.

I've discovered over time that there are many people—like myself—who once could put our trust in the world of empirical, rational science only. Then, a new understanding emerged. It involved a deep transformation of consciousness, one that could no longer deny the reality of the personal spiritual experiences of others. Such experiences pointed to a new understanding of metaphysical reality. If what they were describing and experiencing were true, then the universe was no longer a cold, unfeeling "accident" of nature. This awareness could only lead to a profound reinterpretation of what it meant to be alive and what it meant to be healthy and whole.

Of course the hard-core skeptics and atheists reject all forms of spirituality and therefore relegate religion and personal kinds of spiritual experiences to the world of science fiction and fantasy. A profound turning point in my personal journey was sparked by my exposure to the deeply compelling personal experiences of otherwise normal individuals. Some of them shared very unusual tales that amounted to seeing ghosts and spirits and receiving warnings and intervention from the "other" side. In the process of learning about all these other views of reality, I had to grapple with the nature of those experiences. Were they real? Were they imagined or fabricated? If so, why? Was there anything to be gained by making it up?

The people I initially encountered were not professional psychics or mediums. No one was paying them to share their stories. On the contrary, most had never shared these experiences with others out of fear of appearing foolish—or crazy. Some had even questioned themselves. This was not because *they* didn't believe that their experiences were real. It was actually a function of their awareness of how intolerant our society remains regarding such things. Cultural and societal influences caused them to slip into self-doubt!

Quite a few individuals I met along the way needed to have their personal experiences validated by someone who was objective and respected in the community. I was able to offer those services by playing "psychic courier." I could anonymously relate one person's experience to that of another person whom they had never met. This seemed to satisfy some inner questioning. From my perspective, I was taken by the similar patterns of these experiences that were emerging from the accumulation of such anecdotes. Patterns cannot be ignored—in science or metaphysics. I could see clear, repeatable patterns at work. And they were leading me to profoundly alter my perspective on metaphysical truth.

This chapter includes examples of five types of paranormal experiences. These are just a handful of the many stories I have collected over my years of research. They all reflect the transmission of information by paranormal means. By and large, the experiences I have recorded here all provided the individual involved with knowledge or information that was unusual or "nonordinary." I believe they offer compelling insights for students of metaphysics. And they help validate those unusual moments of psychic experience that so many of us can relate to.

Several examples have already been noted in other portions of this book. Included here are additional events of equal credibility.

I can roughly separate these experiences into categories:

1. The near-death experience (NDE)
2. After-death communications (ADC)
3. Apparitional experiences
4. Reincarnation memories
5. Medium/psychic experiences.

This last category is of a different nature from the others in a significant way. It is not a true "experience." It reflects information being transferred from those on the "other" side to living people, in a paranormal manner. It is powerful and compelling in its own right and may very well offer the participant an insight into the metaphysical mind, body, and spirit reality. But it is not an experience with deeply subjective qualities, as are the others. It must be considered, however, in any metaphysical undertaking, because of the profound implication of its credibility—namely survival of the soul or consciousness after death.

Why is all of this so important? How does this affect our general state of health, or lack thereof? Should we care whether these experiences are real? Absolutely! For me, they have been the fuel for my metaphysical journey. They have kept me moving forward in my own studies and explorations. They have led me to consider the evidence for a deeper, much vaster level of reality. They have offered insight into the question of whether our lives have a higher purpose and how healing can transcend physical and spiritual dimensions. The truth is this: knowledge that life has a deeper meaning is in and of itself a great gift of healing—to all of us.

A STANDARD OF MEASURE

Credibility quotient (CQ) is a term I use to describe the believability of individuals who report personal paranormal and spiritual experiences. I have also referred to these experiences as *unexplained* because of the bias that exists among certain hard-core skeptics who dismiss anything that hints at a spiritual dimension to reality.

The issue of credibility actually involves a broader and quite fascinating topic of how we communicate the subjective feeling of *any* experience to each other. Language is often inadequate or insufficient to transmit the character and quality of our reactions to the events and feelings that characterize our lives.

Certainly, some of us are more articulate than others. We may be more descriptive in our language, offer more examples, or may be more animated in our presentation. But essentially the ability to communicate the essence of an experience often depends on whether the individual with whom we are communicating has had the same or similar kind of experience.

How could I describe what a steak tastes like to someone who has been raised a vegetarian? How can I describe a sunset to someone who is blind? Not easily! So you can just imagine how much more difficult it is to describe a paranormal/spiritual experience to an individual who has not had the same or a similar experience.

The notion of credibility has two distinct but interrelated components. The first is, are the individuals who report these experiences to be believed? In other words, are they hallucinating, or fabricating these experiences in order to garner attention or fame or notoriety for themselves? Are they mentally unbalanced in any way? Are they so desperate to believe in a spiritual dimension to reality that they are grasping for any hint of an experience in order to believe in life after death, in God, in the continuation of consciousness after death?

Second, there is another element to the credibility quotient. Is there any reason to believe in a higher spiritual reality? In God, soul, an afterlife? Is this the private, protected ground of religion alone? What about the personal experiences of ordinary individuals? Should we distrust our own experiences, our encounters with apparitions, with psychics and mediums?

I believe the answer to this conundrum is this: Retain the open-minded skepticism that will guard against unwarranted belief. But be willing to judge the evidence fairly and without prejudice. Be willing to believe what you hear or see if it seems to be the most logical and reasonable answer, even if that answer confuses you and contradicts your previous beliefs.

This discussion can actually lead us into the fascinating but highly complex and controversial nature of consciousness or the mind. How is it possible that we are actually conscious of ourselves as thinking beings? How do we come to believe that an experience is real as opposed to a hallucination or dream?

To the actual individual who has had a deeply personal, highly subjective experience, there is no doubt it is real. This phenomenon has been studied by William James, M.D., the "Father of American Psychology," who wrote about it in *The Varieties of Religious Experiences* in the early part of the twentieth century.

Despite his own lack of such experiences, James offers an objective analysis of them. Like James, I too suffer from what I call *mystic envy*. And like James, I do not let that inadequacy deter me from studying the subject. He was the first to use the concept of *ineffability*—a word which paradoxically means that no words can describe the experience. It is extremely subjective in its impact on the individual involved, and extremely powerful.

Another quality of the experience is *noetic*, meaning a state of knowledge of subtle, spiritual wisdom that is often forgotten or remains vague after the experience is over. Two lesser qualities of the experiences were their relatively short duration and a feeling that the individual is no longer in control of the situation.

Raymond Moody also described the phenomenon in his 1975 landmark book on near-death experience, *Life After Life*. His classic description closely parallels the studies that James refers to. The near-death experience leaves the involved individual with a sense that their experience was totally real, more so than ordinary waking consciousness. Despite arguments that they are the result of hypoxia (lack of oxygen to the brain), the clarity and sharp memory of the experience that does not fade over time, is a powerful argument against the hallucinatory nature of the experience.

One of the most powerful lessons of the NDE is the aftermath. Many individuals note profound alterations in their understanding of the nature of reality: They are more spiritual and less religious, have less interest in material possession and raw ambition, are often more involved with spiritual undertakings, may notice increased psychic abilities, and, finally, may lose the fear of death. Such transformations seem to reflect a genuine and powerfully real spiritual experience.

So with the knowledge that all experiences are personal and subjective, how does one even attempt to judge the experiences of other individuals? This is a significant issue. Yet throughout all my extensive readings and research, I could find no terminology to adequately describe the problem of evaluating the subjective paranormal/spiritual experiences of other individuals. It is essential that we acknowledge that this problem exists—it must be recognized and addressed, otherwise we cannot continue to seek ultimate truth. Otherwise we will continue to ignore or dismiss these powerful, yet deeply personal experiences that are revealing to us something very profound about metaphysical reality—that these experiences are real and that the universe is far more complex and fantastic than science has revealed thus far. Perhaps it is showing us that the world religions may have touched upon a core of spiritual truth after all. Hence I came up with the term *credibility quotient*.

I can remember a time when I completely doubted the validity of a spiritual universe. Until my encounters with individuals who had had personal "unexplained" experiences, I was on the edge of atheism and agnosticism. I had no reason to believe that spiritual belief was anything more than a delusion. It was the credibility of individuals who crossed my path and shared their stories with me that convinced me otherwise. These were people who had nothing to gain, nothing to sell and much to lose by appearing strange and offbeat.

Jen, a nurse, was the first one to move me to open my mind and rethink my position. At first she was completely unwilling to speak to me face to face. I had to call her at night, speak to her over the phone and convince her of my genuine interest in what she had to say. This introduction to someone who was completely sincere and amazingly reluctant to speak was incredibly compelling to me. For the first time in my life I knew that there was something extraordinary and real about what she was describing. My curiosity was stoked. I was hooked.

She had been traumatized by people who had laughed at her stories, had mocked her in her youth. Her courage in sharing them with me paved the way for many more "Jens" to enter my life over time—kind, sincere, otherwise ordinary, honest people who have provided me with the kind of quality of evidence that has motivated me to continue to explore these issues.

I have subsequently heard many compelling stories from other individuals and have cultivated an attitude of deep respect for their personal experiences. Many of these people were tortured by what had happened to them, yet they began to feel comfortable opening up to me.

As I collected more stories I began to see patterns in the experiences, something akin to the process that takes place in the scientific method. I would then share them (anonymously of course) with the other individuals who had seen themselves as somehow different, even as cursed by their own painful revelations. I could perceive a sense of relief when they realized that they were not totally alone. For some, it was a complete revelation to learn that there were many others like them, equally confused and upset, and feeling as if they had to remain silent about what they knew to be true.

My role as psychic courier soon made me known as a sensitive and sympathetic listener. More people came forward to share their stories with me. There was something in our interactions that affected me in a profoundly visceral way. Call it gooseflesh or intuition. There was no doubt that these were *real* and powerful experiences that were being shared with me. I began to develop my own subtle sixth sense about these things. I just knew when someone was telling the truth.

I soon realized, however, that when I would relate these experiences to a third party, a significant degree of the impact of the story was lost. Although the person knew me, but not necessarily the individual I was speaking of, the power of that direct encounter was still somehow diminished. I had received it firsthand. I had been in their presence. I had looked into their eyes as they spoke, watched the expressions on their faces, and heard the tremble in their voice. I could feel the emotion and the truth of these stories, but somehow the essence—the sense of the reality and truth of that experience—wasn't being transmitted to the third party to whom I was now retelling the story.

Although they listened politely, I knew that the third party just didn't seem to get it. The CQ was difficult, if not impossible, to transfer by verbal means alone.

As I continued to accumulate these experiences I soon realized why reading about them in books had little impact on me. The CQ was *tremendously diminished* when reading about someone who was personally unknown to the reader. It became clear to me—in order to comprehend the reality of these "unexplained" experiences, it is crucial to do your own investigations. Nothing short of "doing" your own exploration will do.

HOW TO RAISE YOUR CQ

There is a huge untapped reservoir of unexplained experiences out there. My own journey has provided me with the experiences that have served as my evidence of a spiritual dimension to reality. But you must take charge of your own journey and seek your own evidence.

This may seem extremely challenging, even frightening, to attempt. It is true that it requires an effort, and at first may not yield results. It requires you to take risks, to openly express your interest in such phenomenon and to express your desire to learn more. You must be willing to risk negative comments or funny looks from those who may think that you are a bit "off." You should also be prepared to occasionally observe frightened expressions on the faces of individuals whom you once regarded as rather open-minded and intelligent.

One way to introduce your interest is to share what you have heard (anonymously, of course) with others. Many will at the very least find these stories entertaining. Don't be surprised if they are moved to share some of their own experiences. For many, it may be the first time that they have ever shared them with anyone else!

The CQ of the person sharing the story will convince you of the truth of their experiences. With the proper awareness and an open mind and a sincere attitude you will be surprised how many people will open up and share their spiritual and paranormal experiences.

As you open a new door to reality for yourself, you may do the same for people you meet. Open communication can help others express previously suppressed memories that have been long buried, filed away in some deep recess of the mind labeled "unexplained." It can be extremely healing to release these bottled-up memories and to finally share them with a sympathetic listener. By listening compassionately and with an open mind, you validate the other person's experience and give them "permission" and encouragement to share and to heal.

You might just find you help someone overcome their insecurities and doubts by simply listening respectfully, and even sharing a moment of eye contact that tells them "I know. . . . This is real." In the process you will find more evidence— the fuel for your metaphysical journey.

There are many in our society who feel guilty about having spiritual experiences outside of the bounds of their organized religion. This guilt may deter them from benefiting from the healing nature of these experiences. Your interest and understanding may very well offer them the permission to realize the healing gift such experiences can provide.

CREDIBILITY QUOTIENT CASES

All of the following anecdotes are true. By that statement I mean they were related to me directly by the individuals involved. In every case these were normal, average citizens who had nothing to gain by fabricating any of these stories. Many of them I knew personally; they were patients, friends, hospital staff, and relatives. To protect the privacy of those who opened their lives to me, I have changed their names, but the essential core and points of the experiences remain intact.

As you begin to read these personal anecdotes please be aware of the issue of credibility that I have raised. That is normal and natural. As I have noted, it is actually to be expected. But this merely reflects the CQ. I have categorized them by the "type" of paranormal experience they represent, to help you sort through them with greater ease. In order to come to a fuller, more personal, and more profound understanding of the veracity of these shared experiences, you the reader must be willing to engage in your own surveys of individuals whom you know and trust. In other words, if you truly seek a deeper understanding and validation of this kind of material, then you should be willing to undertake your own metaphysical journey.

These very special stories are the very same that launched my own metaphysical journey from skeptic to meta-physician, and from physician to healer.

Near-Death Experiences

Up the Down Staircase

Sue has been a nurse for at least twenty years. After discovering my interest in the paranormal she sought me out to tell me of an experience that she had shared with few others. It began when she came on duty one morning at 7 A.M. There was a "Code Blue" cardiac arrest in progress and the full team of doctors and nurses were working on an elderly man. He was unconscious and they were prescribing drugs and applying paddles to his chest. They had run out of meds and someone asked Sue to run up to the critical care unit (CCU) and bring some back. She ran up the back stairs, obtained the drugs and returned. She did not really participate in this "code" any further. The patient survived, went to the CCU, and a week or so later returned to the same floor. Sue had not even realized that it was the same patient, but when he saw her he noted, "You were there when they did my cardiac arrest. They didn't have enough medication and you had to run up the back stairs and get some." She was a bit taken aback and immediately thought he was considering some type of lawsuit. "How did you know?" she asked nervously. He laughed, "I was with you when you ran up the stairs!"

Before-Birth Experience

The Baby Dream

The following is an extremely unusual story. It is in effect a before-birth experience told to me by a student in one of my classes at Brookdale College. Jane related to the class a strange dream she had in which she was in a room with a newborn baby. It was a boy and he was crying. Her instinct was to pick him up and try to soothe him. She did, and he seemed to be better. Then she thought she should put him down but realized that no one else was in the room. The baby seemed to be uncomfortable, with distressing abdominal pain. As she was pondering what to do, the baby communicated telepathically with her and told her, "Don't worry, my mommy is waiting for me. I'll see her soon." She awoke from the bizarre dream and told no one about it. A few hours later, a good friend from work called to tell her that her expectant daughter had delivered a baby prematurely, at home. It was a boy, and everything seemed fine. Jane thought a bit about the interesting parallel between her dream and her good friend's new grandson, but didn't say anything other than "I'd like to see your new grandson when you go to visit." A week later, she did visit the newborn and its mom and immediately recognized the baby from her dream. During that visit, Jane noted, the baby did seem to cry a lot and frequently tense his abdomen. But was this so unusual or was she just looking for something? Perhaps, she thought, I'm trying to make my dream fit what's going on with this baby. Perhaps I'm overreacting to a normal situation. The next day she called her friend to see how her baby grandson was doing. Her friend noted that her daughter was a bit concerned because the baby was crying and not eating. She was considering waiting for her next scheduled pediatrician's appointment. Jane advised her friend to tell her daughter not to wait but to bring the baby right in. When her friend questioned her about this opinion she replied, "I don't know but I just have a feeling she shouldn't wait." As it turned out, the pediatrician immediately hospitalized the baby, he had surgery on an incarcerated hernia and did well. Jane later revealed her dream to her skeptical friend who could only reply, "thank you!"

After-Death Communications

The following represent the bulk of the experiences that have been shared with me. Each and every one of them gave me the chills when I first heard them, and, in my estimation, they continue to stand as compelling evidence of the world beyond the five senses.

Wrap Me Up

Sally is a lovely young woman, who is now happily married with several children. She told me this a story about a lover she had years before her marriage, at a time in her life when she was quite young. Apparently her former beloved was older and her family was not in favor of their relationship. But they were deeply in love, and they shared a truly profound and meaningful bond, despite her family's objections to their union. His adoration was evident in a personal expression of endearment that he always used to say to her: "I'd like to wrap you up like a doll and carry you with me."

After several months into the relationship, he developed cancer. His case was advanced and she watched him deteriorate rapidly. It was disheartening to watch his condition worsen, but Sally was with him constantly. Knowing that death was near, he told her that she would someday meet and marry someone else. He promised that when the time was right, he would provide her a sign to let her know it was okay. She protested that she could never love again. He soon died. Although heartbroken, after a year or so she eventually began to date again. She was out on a dinner date one night with a man who really liked her. She liked him too but she was still going through the motions, still numb from the death of the man she loved. Suddenly, the guy she was out with turned to her and said, "I'd like to wrap you up like a doll and carry you with me." Sally said she dropped her fork, turned white, and asked, in a quivering voice, "How could you possibly say that?" Confused, the young man said that he didn't know where that came from. It just popped into his head. Clearly, Sally got her sign from the heavens, as it was promised to her. Subsequently, she married the man and they began a family together.

The Star of David

Miriam and Joe were both patients of mine for many years. Joe, a very funny, jovial guy who often played practical jokes on people, died. A few years later Miriam told me the following story. She and her daughter were driving in the car together and speaking fondly of Joe and what a character he was. Miriam was wearing a Star of David pendant that Joe had given her. It rested on her chest. As she was speaking, she described beginning to feel as if the Star of David pendant was getting warmer. At first she thought it was her imagination but as it got hotter she called out with a laugh, "Joe, cut it out!" When she got out of the car her daughter gasped and pointed out to Miriam that there was a red mark on her chest beneath where the pendant had hung.

Grandpa's Sweater

The following can be classified as an ADC and/or an apparitional encounter.

Joyce was an attractive middle-aged woman, a patient of mine, who related the following experience. She had been close to her father-in-law, Frank, who had died about six months before this unusual experience. One night she awoke to find him standing at the foot of her bed, bathed in a pale light. He was smiling and looked years younger. Although he was somewhat transparent she could see clearly what he was wearing and described his checked sweater. She made a mental note of it, right down to and including the color. She fell back to sleep and in the morning wondered whether she had dreamt the whole episode. She had no intention of telling anyone. That morning her teenage daughter came down to breakfast—very agitated. She described how she had awoken in the middle of the night to see Grandpa standing at the foot of her bed smiling. When Joyce asked what he was wearing, her daughter described having seen the exact same sweater.

Sports Channel

Sylvia is a lovely elderly woman who is nearly 80, but appears much younger. I usually see her in my office every year of so for her gastrointestinal problems. I could tell during one visit that she had been under considerable stress but assumed it was regarding her elderly husband's health. I was shocked when she informed me that her adult son had committed suicide about nine months earlier. She was upset on so many levels, unaware that he had been so depressed over his personal matters. She related to me several experiences that occurred about three months after he died. She stated that although her son was an incredible sports fan and watched it on TV constantly, she was absolutely *not interested* in sports. She did her ironing late at night, in the basement with the TV on to keep her company but the channel was always tuned to the *Tonight Show*. One night she went to bed, late as usual; her husband awoke before her the next day. When she came down to breakfast, her husband, who got up before her, remarked that he had found the TV on in the basement. Sylvia had *thought* that she had turned it off, but acknowledged that perhaps she hadn't. Several weeks later, she was again up late at night, ironing and watching TV (anything but sports). This time she specifically *recalled* turning the TV off. But the next morning again her husband noted that the TV had been on when he awoke. Now she was getting a bit upset because she clearly recalled turning it off. Several weeks went by and she was again doing her ironing in the basement. She definitely turned the TV off and went to bed after her husband. This time she couldn't sleep and got up before her husband. She found the TV on—and it was on the sports channel. She began to sob and her husband told her for the first time that every time he found the TV on, it was on the sports channel.

Message in the Sand

Patti works in the endoscopy department at the hospital, helping to clean our scopes after our procedures. She related the following story. Her father died and she and her sister traveled to Cape Cod for the funeral. The day before, the two sisters went to their father's favorite beach. It was his favorite place to fish. It was a cold March day—dreary, drizzling, and overcast. It was a Tuesday and had rained the night before. No one was around. The beach was desolate and empty. As she was leaving the beach she said out loud, "Daddy, I love you." She and her sister got into the car and started to drive off. Her sister stopped the car and pointed to a nearby sand dune. In letters about a foot high there were clear letters in the sand. There was a heart shape preceded by the letter *I* and followed by the letter *U* and the number 2. It was a clear message, "I love you two." And it was without doubt a response to Patti's call. She took a picture with her cell phone and showed it to me. It was quite clear.

A Beep from Beyond

Carmella is an operating room nurse. She described to me a conversation she had previously had with her favorite aunt, Marie. They were both at the funeral of another relative and were chatting about the possibility of life after death. Marie said that since she was quite a bit older, in all likelihood she would die first. She promised that, if possible, she would too offer Carmella a sign if there was "life after death." They both laughed it off at the time and Carmella gave no more thought to it. Several years later, Carmella was "on-call" to the operative room. This meant she could sleep at home but needed to be available by telephone for any emergency cases. She always carried a beeper as a backup. Around 4 A.M. one morning, her beeper went off. Alarmed, she asked her husband to make sure that the phone was not off the hook, then checked the beeper. She didn't recognize the extension as a hospital number. Her husband told her that it was probably a mistake and to go back to sleep. She slipped back into bed and into a deep sleep. But suddenly she bolted out of bed yelling, "That number on the beeper, that's her birthday. I bet Aunt Marie is dead." Two hours later the phone rang. It was true.

Radio Broadcast from Beyond

Art is a long-time patient of mine who has shared many of his paranormal experiences with me. This one is particularly compelling. Both his parents had died relatively young. His mother, however, had committed suicide. Trying to process his pain, Art got into drugs, as well as meditation. One day he was concentrating on his mother and she appeared to him in his apartment. He asked if she was with his dad, her husband, and she replied that she wasn't ready to be at his level (implying that because of the suicide, she had more lessons to learn on the other side). Art then asked her for some sign or evidence that she had been there so he could call his sister, Sally. She was upset and angry with Art for his lifestyle and the two rarely spoke. His mother told him to turn on the radio after she "left." He did and heard a popular song at the time, "You and Me Against the World" by Helen Reddy. It meant very little to him. He called his sister anyway, and she was still too annoyed to want to speak to him. Before she could hang up, he told her about the "visitation" from Mom and the radio message. When he mentioned the song, the phone went dead. His sister became speechless, so her husband wanted to know what Art had said. The sister got back on and said, "Didn't you know what that song meant to Mom and Dad?" Art admitted that he didn't. "They would both sing it together when they came over to my house!"

Uncle Sal's Special Shirt

Joyce was a nurse from Staten Island who related this story to me shortly after the attack on the World Trade Center on 9/11. Her uncle Sal, who worked for the Port Authority, died that day. They had been very close and Sal was only a few years older than Joyce. A few weeks later she had a very vivid dream in which Sal was present at a typical Sunday afternoon Italian family picnic. He looked great and the only unusual feature was the loud Hawaiian shirt he was wearing. Apparently Sal was into Ralph Lauren and Calvin Klein shirts, so this Hawaiian shirt was a particularly strange aspect of the dream. Joyce could clearly see that this was a black shirt with pink, yellow, and blue flowers. The next morning she called her father, Sal's brother, to discuss the dream and the shirt. Her father was stunned. "How could you know about that shirt?" he exclaimed. He had found that exact shirt in Sal's SUV, which was located in a garage after 9/11. Her dad had been the only one who knew about the shirt and Sal's plan for a vacation in Hawaii.

The Dedicated Nurse

Jen was the source of many of the stories of spiritual and paranormal phenomenon from my early days of exploration and collecting material. She had an older friend named Betty, also a nurse, who had been a confidant, mentor, and friend. They had gotten particularly close after Jen's husband had died. Betty was rather old-fashioned and happened to be extremely petite. Her whole life was nursing and she was extremely dedicated. She insisted on wearing an old-fashioned nursing hat and pin, of which she was extremely proud. Betty unexpectedly died one night while working. The other nurses found her on the floor in the midst of performing the role she loved best in life. Several months later, Jen reported that it was an incredibly busy night, which meant very sick patients. Some were being transferred to the intensive care unit (ICU), others were going for emergency surgery. An elderly man at the end of the hall rang his bell for water. Jen intended to see him but got caught up in all the chaos. It wasn't until several hours later that she remembered his request. She ran down the hall to find him asleep. He woke up and when she apologized about the water, he said, "Oh, don't worry. This other nurse came by and helped me. She wore an old-fashioned cap and pin. She was so tiny that she didn't have to bend over when she gave me the water."

Smoke Signals

Dr. M. is an anesthesiologist originally from Thailand. When his older brother was dying, he returned to his homeland to be with him. He recalled leaving his brother's room to take a walk with one of his nieces. He carried his brother's cell phone with him. Several minutes later, as he was walking, he was overwhelmed by the smell of the kind of incense you would encounter at a Buddhist temple. He asked his niece if she smelled it—she didn't. Later when they returned to the hospital they discovered that the brother had died, around the same time that Dr. M. smelled the incense. Later he was told that in the Thai Buddhist tradition, this was a way that those who died notified their family. About an hour later his brother's cell phone rang. On the other end was another niece. When Dr. M. inquired as to why she called on that line, she replied, "That phone called me!"

My British Grandpa

Carolyn worked in one of the hospitals whose staff I was on in Old Bridge, New Jersey. Her job was that of patient assistant. She told me about an incredibly vivid dream she had one night. In the dream, she had a visit from her English grandfather. She explained that her father was an American GI, her mother an English woman, and they had met during World War II. She was conceived in England but born in the United States. She had very little contact with her English grandfather because of the high costs of travel. They would correspond by letter and an occasional phone call. Carolyn was aware that as she was his first grandchild, he had always wanted her to visit. She described that one night, during an amazingly vivid dream, it was if the ceiling of her bedroom "opened up" and her grandfather was there. He looked well but kept shaking his head and asking, "Why didn't you visit? Why didn't you visit?" He was standing with his hands on his hips and was wearing glasses with old-fashioned frames. Carolyn had never seen them before. The next morning she called her mother to describe the dream, his stance, and the glasses. She confirmed that he used to stand that way and that she recalled him wearing glasses with that type of frame. They ended the conversation in a joyful mood and hung up the phone. Fifteen minutes later the phone rang. Her mother was in tears when she told Carolyn, "I just got the call, Grandpa died last night."

Cosmic Law and Order

Jane was another patient of mine for many years, and also a student in my metaphysics classes. Her husband Ralph died after a long bout with stomach cancer. She was able to care for him at home with hospice support. They would sometimes watch the medium John Edward on TV and had discussed the possibility of life after death. Jane asked Ralph to give her a sign. "But don't scare me," she told him. When his time came, he passed over. She described an incident that occurred during his wake. About eight people were at her home and they all heard—through the baby monitor that had been in his bedroom—sounds of his favorite TV show, Law and Order. Jane asked her son-in-law to go into the room and turn the TV off. He came back pale and shaking and reported that the TV had not been on and the baby monitor had not even been plugged in.

Papa's Cane

The following is both an ADC and an apparitional experience. (In effect, apparitional experiences fit into this same category.) This is the experience of Dr. T., an anesthesiologist from Pakistan. He reluctantly shared this experience with me after hearing that I was open to discussing the topic. He was in this country studying for his exams. It was extremely late at night and he had not been in Pakistan for months. Suddenly his father appeared in his apartment walking with a cane. He had never seen his father with a cane. His father said something to the effect of "It's my time." Then he disappeared and Dr. T. assumed he had been hallucinating from fatigue. He fell asleep and a few hours later the phone rang. It was from Pakistan announcing that his father was gravely ill. He was determined to return home but was told that his father had wanted him to stay and complete his exams. The next day he was told that his father died. He couldn't get back to Pakistan for a few weeks. When he finally did and entered his family's home he saw the exact same cane. When he questioned his mother she admitted that his father had needed to use a cane in the few weeks before his death.

Miguel's Appearance

This story comes from a woman named Rose who works in my endoscopy center. Rose also works at the hospital, which is where she met Pablo, an elderly Hispanic man who was her patient. He had suffered a heart attack and was very weak. One morning he told her that his son Miguel came into his room late at night. He was afraid that he would get into trouble because it was after visiting hours. Later that morning Rose heard that his son Miguel had died the night before in a car accident and had been in the ICU of the same hospital. His family was afraid to tell Pablo because of his bad heart.

The Twirling Ring

The following is primarily an apparitional experience by a psychically gifted individual. Marilyn worked in the hospital as a unit secretary. She was as upset as everyone else when she learned that the twenty-year-old daughter of one of the staff nurses, Janet, had died tragically in a car accident. She knew Janet fairly well but had never met her daughter. She described driving up Janet's home the night of the wake and feeling uneasy about going in. Marilyn has experienced a lifetime of psychic intuitions and insights that had nearly always proven accurate. She entered Marilyn's home, saw photographs of the deceased daughter and immediately recognized her standing amid a crowd appearing uneasy, and anxious. She appeared somewhat transparent and no one else seemed to notice her. Many people come to their own funerals. Individuals who die suddenly, without warning, can often appear restless, dazed, and out of sorts, because the soul is shocked out of the body. Of significance to Marilyn was the observation that the daughter was quickly twirling one of her rings around her finger. She left shortly and vowed to speak with Janet in several weeks, when some of the initial shock had worn off. She finally did and made mention of "seeing" her daughter at her own wake. Janet seemed shocked and disbelieving, but when Marilyn mentioned seeing her twirling the ring of her finger, Janet broke down in tears. Yes, indeed, that was her habit when she was under stress.

Blond Apparition I

The following is an apparitional experience that occurred to Kathleen, a nurse I work with. She and her husband decided to renovate their kitchen at home. It was an older house with previous owners and when they pulled away the cabinets they found a drawing that had slipped behind. It was rather old and partially faded but appeared to be a birthday drawing apparently from a young girl to her father. They took the drawing and laid it out on the table and left it there. Later, Kathleen and her sister were resting in their living room when they saw a young blond-haired girl climb the steps to the upstairs level. Believing that it was her daughter, Kathleen called out to her. The girl did not turn around. She called louder, and her daughter answered—from another room. The next day Kathleen spoke with neighbors who recalled that in the past a young blond girl had died in that home from leukemia. She subsequently located the father of that young girl and mailed him the drawing. Kathleen did not mention the blond girl on the staircase.

Blond Apparition II

Geraldine, who worked in my endoscopy center, had had many psychic and spiritual experiences throughout her life. She grew up in a home that was at least one hundred years old. She recalled having a mysterious blond-haired playmate who would appear from behind some furniture; the girl wore an old-fashioned dress. Years later, her much younger step-brother slept in that same room. Except for her own Mother, she had never discussed her childhood experiences with him, or anyone else for that matter. Spontaneously, he one day described seeing the same exact little girl with the same dress to his mother.

The Exorcism and the Singing Bird

The following comes from my first cousin, Charles, a devout skeptic. He shared this story with no one until he discovered that I was open and interested in such phenomena. He described the time when, as a film student at NYU, he and several other students were given the opportunity to assist one of their professors on a film he was shooting. It was to take place on a small farm in upstate New York that was apparently haunted. The film was to be about an exorcism. Although all the students were extremely skeptical, they realized it was, at the very least, a weekend out of the city. As they were setting up the shoot, the young children who had recently moved into the home invited them into the one bedroom that seemed to be the center of "activity." It was a decidedly "cold" room, and a parrot was kept there. The kids claimed that the parrot would speak nonstop until it was placed there. Charles and his fellow students were extremely cynical, doubting that the bird ever made noise. Later a psychic and a minister showed up to begin the proceedings. The cameras were rolling. The psychic confirmed that the site of paranormal activity was the "cold" bedroom. The rite of exorcism began in that cold bedroom at midnight. After what seemed like several hours with many incantations and prayers, the minister let out a loud shriek and fell backwards, passing out. Everyone became alarmed. Immediately, however, the room became much warmer and the parrot began to sing. In a state of shock, all the students and crew went down to the kitchen. Then someone noticed—all the clocks in the house and everyone's watch had stopped at exactly 3 A.M.

The Smoking Medium

This is an exceeding strange tale involving Carolyn, again. Her husband had died and several months later she was sitting outside of the hospital in the smoking area. A patient showed up with an intravenous (IV) pole in one hand

and a cigarette in the other. Although Carolyn had never seen this woman before in her life, she took one look at Carolyn and proceeded to describe a middle-aged tall man with salt-and-pepper hair. It was clear to Carolyn that it was her deceased husband. The woman claimed that he wanted to express his love and thank her for placing her photo in the inside pocket of his suit before he was laid to rest. Carolyn said that no one knew that. She had privately done it when no one was around. This stranger then proceeded to say that her husband wanted to make sure she did not forget about the "green metal box." Carolyn told the woman that she had no idea what she was talking about, but the woman with the IV pole was quite insistent about remembering the "green metal box." Later Carolyn spoke with one of her daughters about the strange encounter. When she mentioned the "green metal box," her daughter immediately responded: "Yes . . . Daddy had left a green metal box with money for you. You're supposed to buy some jewelry with it."

Just in the Knick of Time

Irene was a student in several of my Brookdale College courses. She related to the class the story of having tragically lost her son to brain cancer at a very young age. Some time afterward, she was driving down a road headed toward a green light. Out of nowhere, her deceased son appeared next to her in the front seat, yelling for her to "stop the car! stop the car!" She was understandably taken aback but stopped the car, expecting to get hit from behind. Instead a car came racing through the red light. It would have hit and possibly killed her. She felt certain that she had been saved by her deceased son.

Hearing Her Name Called Saves Her Life

A parallel story comes from Beth, one of my patients. Knowing my interest in such phenomena she described sitting at a red light waiting for it to turn green. Just as it was about to do so, she turned her head to the left because she heard her name being called from the back seat. No one was there, of course, but as she turned she saw a car barreling through the red light into the intersection that she would have entered.

Reincarnation and the Council of Elders

Marvin was one of the few male students in one of my classes at Brookdale College in metaphysics. After listening to several students express their experiences, he told about his past-life memory. His background was important to know. Born in Italy, he came to this country as a young boy. However, he always had a "memory" of coming from the Midwest of the United States. He recalls vividly growing up on a farm, and when World War II breaks out, all of his friends signed up to fight. He recalls a farewell party, getting on a large gray ship to travel with other soldiers to Europe. He was stationed in either France or Germany. His recollection is vivid: He can smell the battlefield. He's dug in with the other GIs.

Incoming artillery shells are getting closer and closer. There is a flash of light. Boom. He knows that he is dead. Afterward, he appears with several other souls in front of a "Council of Elders" to discuss his previous life and whether he met his goals. He recalls protesting that his life was over too soon and that we wanted to back into the Army. He is told that he has to wait, but that eventually it will happen. Marvin, born in Italy, would come to the States and eventually sign up for the Army to fulfill his mission. Of considerable interest to me was that Marvin had never read the works of Michael Newton, who refers to the Council of Elders in all of his books involving the reports of his clients under deep hypnosis. When I asked Marvin to read and report back, he did so and was quite shaken. The book was very real to him, he said.

Consulting Mediums

Why would I consider the question of mediums as essential to this issue of metaphysical reality, and how does it relate to the question of health and healing? Quite frankly it comes down to exploring the fundamental issues of what is real. If what mediums claim to do is real, then we should all recognize the futility of most of our fears. If there is continuation of the soul after death, if our loved ones are never truly gone, if our physical existence in this lifetime, in this physical body, is a temporary state of being, then we need to incorporate this wisdom into our concepts of what it means to be alive. We need to allow the truth of the survival of the soul to sink into our consciousness. It can transform our daily lives. We know how the quality of our daily lives can be impacted by our state of mind. This is only compounded by the scientific evidence of the mind–body connection. How much of our agitation, worry, despair, and concern would be lifted by a true awareness of the survival of our soul? Happier, less-stressed individuals not only experience a better quality of life but experience better physical health as well. Reduced stress means a more competent and capable immune system, lower blood pressure, longer life.

I invite you to examine the following experiences, ponder them, and seek confirmation for yourselves. I am a believer who is working with a medium who has demonstrated extraordinary abilities. There are no board certifications or state licenses to confirm the validity of someone claiming such unusual gifts. Like choosing an attorney or physician, it may ultimately be a matter of personal references.

The field has long been plagued by charges of fakery and fraud and clearly there have been many who have been found guilty as charged. But as the following anecdotes will hopefully demonstrate, there are individuals who demonstrate knowledge of facts and events that defy common sense and rational logic.

Boris, the Medium from Odessa

A Russian medium, Boris, was particularly on target with many people I knew. We first came to meet him through Jane. Jane became aware of his presence through a complex sequence of events. A sister of a friend of Jane's was in Cape May on vacation when Boris approached her in a small food store. He explained that he was a medium and before she could walk away, he proceeded to tell her that her dead lover would not leave Boris alone until he spoke with her. After a few minutes, she was convinced that Boris was for real. She had a reading with him the next day. In the session, a message came through for a "Jane." This woman knew few women named Jane, including her sister's friend Jane, who apparently had two deceased sisters who needed to get through to her. Eventually Jane met Boris and described a most incredible reading with him. He was so specific that Jane said to me, "Before I met him I wasn't sure I believed in life after death, now I know it!" Jane arranged for many others to have readings with Boris. Some were better than others. One in particular involved a nurse Elizabeth whose husband had died. She had kept a box of his private items that she could not discard. Boris literally named every object in that box. Elizabeth was stunned.

Ray, the Upstate Medium

I had an opportunity to have an hour reading with a medium, originally from New York City who now lives in Upstate New York area. This occurred about a month after my mother died. He accurately mentioned her brother who had died first, then absolutely mentioned her first name, "Millie." This is not the most common of names and this was how she was known. He followed this up with other rather personal confirmations, including the prediction that I would be the author of a book.

Artie, the Coolest Medium

My personal favorite is Artie, who has become a friend as well. My initial personal reading with him involved three of my family members who had died. He so accurately described their personalities and their familiar expressions that it would have been impossible to substitute one reading for another. I knew that he knew nothing about me that first time. I also knew that this was not a "cold" reading in which generalities are thrown out and desperately grasped. Subsequently, Artie and his "Artie Parties" become well known in the area. Some of his readings involving others were even more astounding.

He did several readings with my office staff. My office manager, Wanda, showed him pictures of both her deceased mother and her husband. Artie mentioned that "Tom is going to move." Wanda had just spoken to Tom, her son, the morning of the reading and their conversation did concern a question of whether or not he should change his residence. No way that Artie could have known that! When gazing at her husband's picture, Artie said, "He wants me to say the word 'dangerous'—does that mean anything to you?" Indeed it did. "Dangerous" may have been the first word her children learned growing up. It was a family joke because it was applied to everything.

I was a witness to a reading Artie conducted with a woman who works as a drug company representative. She brought pictures of both her deceased grandparents. Artie asked, "Who is Cecilia?" The woman responded that she didn't know anyone by that name. He then broke into song and began to sing "Ce-Cecilia, you're breaking my heart," the Simon and Garfunkel song. She smiled and then immediately recalled that her grandparents always played that song when she was visiting their house.

At another time, Artie performed perhaps the most incredible reading I have ever heard of. It is particularly powerful and compelling to me because I know Artie and the young woman, Mandy, who had the reading with him. She is an employee in my medical office and I know her quite well. It seems as if Tuesday night (before her Saturday reading) she was in bed and thinking about her deceased grandmother. She reported later that she felt her grandmother's presence up in her room near the ceiling. She didn't exactly *see* her but was certain about the *feeling*. She never told anyone. And frankly, she even questioned herself the next day. Saturday arrived and she sat down with Artie for her reading. He stared at a picture of the grandmother and said, "Your grandmother says she was in your bedroom Tuesday night up near the ceiling." Mandy was totally stunned, speechless. I have had the opportunity to repeatedly question her about the initial experience and about her reading with Artie. There is not doubt that both occurred the way I have described them.

FINDING YOUR OWN PATH TO PSYCHIC PHENOMENON

William James, M.D., physician, psychologist, meta-physician, and psychic researcher explored the question of the *validity* of the medium experience. He understood the bias against accepting the extraordinary claims implicit in the work that mediums presumably do. He also made a crucial point of emphasizing that all mediums did not have to be truly gifted in order to validate that there are many who are quite gifted. This concept holds true for people in any profession. For example, some doctors happen to be more gifted than others, just as certain nurses seem to have more of a healing touch than others.

It might take some time to let in—and adjust your listening to be able to hear—the kernels of truth in the stories people share about their experiences with this phenomenon. Take one step at a time and one story at a time. You never know what an open mind may bring your way. At stake is nothing less than a radically powerful understanding of the nature of reality and our place within it. From the context of this perspective, transformation and healing can follow.

APPENDIX: ADDITIONAL INSIGHTS FROM
THE CREDIBILITY QUOTIENT

This Appendix provides readers with additional scientific information related to Part IV, "The Credibility Quotient." In his book *The "God" Part of the Brain*,

Matthew Alper offers convincing arguments that mankind seems to be genetically predisposed to religious belief. He acknowledges, as do nearly all anthropologists and psychologists, that belief in a spiritual reality is universal. There is little debate about this characteristic of all human societies from across the globe.

He refers to the work of Andrew Newberg and Eugene D'Aquili at the Nuclear Medicine division at the University of Pennsylvania. They used SPECT (single positron emission computed tomography) to demonstrate that spiritual/mystical experiences are located within physical areas and structures of the brain. Alper's conclusion is that *there is no reason to conclude that a spiritual dimension to reality actually exists.* He says it is a figment of mankind's collective and personal imagination based upon certain common human neural processes.

Most interesting to me, however, is that Newberg and D'Aquili come to an entirely different conclusion. In their book *Why God Won't Go Away,* they study the biology of belief by scanning Buddhist monks and Franciscan nuns at prayer. The SPECT scans revealed similar findings: a reduced activity of the orientation association area, OAA. Such a finding coincided with the mystical experience of oneness with the universe, a classic description of the mystical experiences.

Newberg points to the subjective nature of reality that has been debated by meta-physicians of all types (philosophers, theologians, scientists) since the dawn of human consciousness. To Alper's (and other skeptics') assertion that mystical and spiritual experiences are all "in the brain"—Newberg points out that "all" experiences are "in the brain."

Alper and other skeptical neuroscientists often point to a scan and make the point that a spiritual experience is merely the result of activation of certain areas in the brain. To their interpretation, this invalidates the experience as truly spiritual, instead demonstrating to their satisfaction that it is a physical reaction that can be scanned and photographed. They can point to specific areas on a SPECT scan and, in their minds, dismiss the spiritual component by pointing out where it occurs in the brain.

Newberg, however, points out that just because science can identify a specific scan pattern for spiritual experience, this does not invalidate the reality of those experiences. More important, this does not invalidate any claims of a higher spiritual reality. It merely reflects where in the human brain such experiences are perceived.

He also contends quite clearly that if a SPECT scan is performed of someone eating an apple pie, it will reveal a distinctive pattern reflecting neural activity within the brain as well. From my perspective, a scan that reveals the location of this experience does not invalidate the *truth* of the experience. That individual really did eat some pie! Similarly, just because a deeply spiritual experience was located to specific areas of the brain, this does not invalidate the metaphysical reality of such experiences occurring.

Newberg and D'Aquili offer a fascinating analysis of subjective experiences, a conceptual basis for evaluating "truth," and state that each individual can judge the relative reality of their own experiences. In other words, someone may *believe* that a dream is real during the dream itself. When they awaken, however, they will be able to compare the sense of reality of the dream state with the awake state. Unless they are on some kind of mind-altering drug, they can clearly evaluate the awake state as being more real than the dream state. This test of relative reality can be applied to mystical and paranormal states of consciousness. The results, however, are strikingly profound. When comparing mystical or paranormal states of consciousness with the awake state, there is nearly universal agreement among individuals that the mystical state is more real than the awake state!

Newberg and D'Aquili conclude that this higher mystical state that they refer to as the "Absolute Unitary Being" is the absolute reality, one that transcends what we ordinarily refer to as the objective and subjective worlds.

This is a compelling and fascinating conclusion from two highly professional students (scholars?) of neuroscience. It should be considered when investigating the claims of ordinary individuals who have had such experiences. One needs to listen carefully to their experiences and consider them seriously.

Part V

Spiritual View on the Nature of Life: Inspirations from Kabbalah and Buddha

We are not human beings having a spiritual experience, we are spiritual being having a human experience.

—Pierre Teilhard de Chardin, Jesuit priest, paleontologist

13

Born Again: Reincarnation and Karma

Being born twice is no more remarkable than being born once.

—Voltaire

The soul casts off and puts on bodies as a man might take off old clothes and put on new ones.

—Bhagavad-Gita

Many religious and spiritual traditions throughout history, and around the world, have understood the meaning of reincarnation. Reincarnation refers to the belief that souls return numerous times into different physical bodies in order to learn and evolve spiritually. It remains a core belief in many of the world's traditions today.

It has always been an aspect of Hinduism and Buddhism. It is also part of the Sikh, Shinto, Jain, and Pagan point of view, as well as many other earth-based religions. Even Judaism's Kabbalistic perspective recognizes it. Islam has proscriptions against it and Christianity finally rejected it several hundreds years after the death of Jesus.

The concept of reincarnation is usually linked to the notion of karma. The soul is the immortal aspect of the human being, and the carrier of karma accrued over many lifetimes. Each new incarnation into a physical body provides the soul with opportunities to either spiritually advance, remain stagnant or, even, regress.

Karma is the sum total of all one's deeds, good and bad.

The evolution of the soul in each lifetime depends upon the freewill choices made by the individual. For example, we make decisions in everyday life that can prevent the soul from evolving—such as engaging in self-destructive behavior or participating in activities that hurt others. We also make decisions that bring us "good karma," such as taking care of our own bodies, minds, and spirits as well as acts of compassion, charity, and kindness toward others.

Each lifetime is a new chance to "get it right," so to speak. We are constantly presented with challenges, large and small, that are opportunities to move our souls forward. If we ignore or avoid these opportunities, they do not go away. Rather, we can look forward to dealing with them in the *next* lifetime ... and then some. The goal is eventual freedom from the cycle of reincarnation and a blissful unification with the ultimate Source or God. There are a multitude of variations on the "theme" of reincarnation and karma. Hinduism believes the same soul incarnates over and over again, paying karmic debts as it goes along. It teaches that when faced with a huge conflict, we must honor karmic duty. Hindus believe karma helps create our destiny in each lifetime and some see it as being out of their hands. But there are prayers and worship services individuals can partake in, designed to lessen the impact of karma in one's current lifetime. One can even "hire" spiritually advanced yogis to help pray your way to a ticket to *nirvana*, or *moksha*, liberation from the cycle of births.

Buddhism, which evolved as a reaction and resistance to Hinduism, denies the existence of a persistent soul. Instead that tradition speaks of an evolving, ever-changing consciousness that somehow still carries karmic debt from life to life.

The earth-based religion, Wicca, teaches that reincarnation is the instrument through which our souls are perfected, as well. They believe that before the soul enters the body, it chooses what kind of life it will have, selecting experiences that will provide the lessons and insights the soul needs to grow. They also believe strongly in what might be called "instant karma." Followers are taught to walk a path of high integrity and to harm none. The belief is that the energy we put out in the world comes back to us threefold, good or bad.

There have been attempts to study reincarnation in a scientific way. Ian Stevenson, MD, has been documenting case studies from children who remember past lives in extraordinary ways and he has produced compelling evidence in his studies. For example, young children would be brought dozens of miles from their homes to visit homes they had never seen, yet they could describe the location of rooms and objects and claimed to remember them from their previous life. They would address adults in these homes, who were the adult children of deceased parents, as if they were still their children. It was reported that these children recognized family-specific events and relationships that only the deceased could have known. It was concluded that these children had retained knowledge of a prior lifetime in this village.

There is also a huge body of work in the area of past life regression, which is a way to bring to the surface past-life memories while under deep hypnosis. The work of Dr. Brian Weiss and Dr. Michael Newton is particularly compelling and enlightening. Each began as a traditionally trained skeptic and agnostic. Weiss was a psychiatrist who risked his professional reputation as Chairman of the Department at the University of Miami. Newton was a Ph.D. in psychology.

Newton found himself directing his patients into deep hypnotic states in which they described their existence in between their past lives. After nearly forty years of performing hypnotic regressions on over seven thousand patients, and compiling their testimonies, he formulated a picture of the between-life state of the soul that has become a classic definition of where the soul goes after physical death. He formulated this based on thousands of consistently similar descriptions from individual patients under deep hypnosis.

This view of the afterlife reveals an environment in which souls recognize each other from past lives, and hang out together and critique or compliment each other over their ability to overcome their previous life challenges. As in the near-death experience, the soul is conscious immediately after death but cannot communicate with the living. A journey to a place where souls congregate is described as a homecoming of sorts. Eventually a meeting before a Council of Elders, with a discussion of the karma from the past life, and plans for future incarnations, are planned. Karma accumulates but rebirth is not automatic. Free will exists even for the soul after death. He has published three books over a fifteen-year period, which confirms his original theories, and I highly recommend you read them for yourself (*Journey of Soul*, *Destiny of Souls*, and *Life Between Life*).

In my own research I came across many individuals with personal experiences that were highly suggestive of reincarnation. It was through hearing their stories that I began to formulate my personal understanding of this aspect of the nature of reality—that the soul never dies.

Sometimes we return to a new body, yet we may, at times, retain memories or glimpses from lives past. Less obvious signs of a past life may include specific talents or interests in certain cultures, countries, or traditions that could not be explained away by one's childhood upbringing. Some people actively pursue these glimpses because they feel it gives them a head start on cleaning up old karma. Others very organically stumble into experiences and wisdom that tells them they have lived before.

The question often arises, "If this is all true, why don't we all recall our past lives?" I believe the answer to this is demonstrated by the children in Ian Stevenson's research. They recall details of their past life, and confuse that life with their present one: they are burdened with memories that hinder their participation in the new life, which has its own challenges to face and overcome.

Amanda is a nurse I have worked with for years at the hospital. I know her mother and father as well. She is a completely sensible, down-to-earth, and reliable witness of life's events. She has described her husband Gary (a retired police officer who has also been my patient) as someone with a passion for Irish music and a fascination with the Civil War.

When Gary was on the force he once arrested a "perp" whom he had never met before, but who was well known to the other cops—and they all considered him to be a bit "weird." Gary, however, discovered that he was perhaps clairvoyant. This fellow took one look at Gary and the first thing he blurted out was, "You love Irish music and you were *in* the Civil War!"

Apparently Gary's mouth flew open and he was speechless. There is little that anyone can say in response to hearing such a story, other than, "Wow! That's weird." Yet the fact that the two men met was not a coincidence. Perhaps Gary needed to receive such a jolt of metaphysical awareness at that time in his life. Just perhaps it helped him to explain the why and what-for of his own journey. Whether or not this encounter propelled him toward a more spiritual path remains to be seen. It was certainly an eye-opener for him. Cindy is another person with a story that, at first, seemed so hard to swallow. She had shared multiple unexplained experiences in dreaming about her deceased father, so I was familiar with the fact that she was "tuned in." One time she told me about a recurrent nightmare that had plagued her most of her life. It took place, she knew, in the Warsaw ghetto in Poland during World War II. Cindy is Polish Catholic, so she was unaware that the victims of the Warsaw ghetto had been Jewish.

She described being chased with her young blond daughter through the streets of the ghetto by Nazi soldiers. She could describe exactly what she looked like, what she was wearing, what her young daughter looked like as well. The dream was terrifying and she would always awaken just as she was trying to hide her daughter inside a building, under the stairs. Cindy would awaken from this dream sweating and crying.

One day, the subject of dreams came up at a family gathering. She felt moved to share this dream with her siblings. It was the first time she'd ever mentioned it to family. As she related her experience, her younger sister began to sob. Recovering from the sudden outburst, she told Cindy, "I keep having the same exact dream, but in the dream . . . I am the daughter."

This brought a sudden sense of recognition and clarity to Cindy, because, as she related to me, "For some reason, I have always regarded my younger sister more like a daughter than sibling." Neither of them had that dream again.

It gave me chills when I heard this, somehow confirming in my very being that it was all true. What does this mean? I believe it shows us that deeply personal experiences of ordinary individuals can help illuminate an incredibly profound aspect of the metaphysical nature of reality—namely, that reincarnation is for real!

Many schools of metaphysical belief and practice agree that reincarnation is part of our reality here on earth. A metaphysical view of being born again . . . and again . . . helps us make sense of our lives. It would explain why life is full of difficult challenges—why else bother to incarnate? We may question the wisdom of our souls in accepting the pain that we must endure. For example, you may wonder why would a soul sign on for a lifetime in which destiny will lead it to lose a child in war, become financially ruined, be unlucky in love, die from a terrible illness, suffer through loss and tragedy?

Michael Newton himself provides this answer, "You were not given your body by a chance of nature. . . . Thus you are not a victim of circumstance. . . . We must not lose sight of the idea that we accepted this sacred contract of life; this means the roles we play on Earth are actually greater than ourselves."

That which you suffer from in any one lifetime, you learn for eternity. Our suffering is not in vain—at least not for those who face life's dramas and obstacles with courage, optimism, and the determination to move on.

Reincarnation and karma may account for a life that seems like one long "survival training program," yet it also provides the context and opportunity for the soul to achieve spiritual advancement and healing.

14

Death as a Transition, Not a Tragedy

There is only a single supreme idea on earth: the concept of immortality of the human soul; all other profound ideas by which men live are only an extension of it.

—Fydor Dostoevsky, writer

The conquest of fear of death is the recovery of life's joy. One can experience an unconditional affirmation of life only when one has accepted death, not as contrary to life but as an aspect of life.

—Joseph Campbell, PhD, writer/anthropologist

So, who *is* afraid of them ghosts? Please confess right now—isn't the question about life after death the most basic, most common, most fear-inspiring metaphysical issue that confronts us all?

Do we exist for this lifetime only? Do we continue in some conscious form for eternity? Do we come back again in another physical form? Do we cease to exist upon the death of our bodies? These are questions that do not discriminate between rich or poor, simple or sophisticated. Just the thought that we, and everyone we love, will cease to exist is enough to shake us to our very core. It taps into our deepest, most powerful fears—our own mortality as well as that of those we love and cherish the most.

DOES DEATH EQUATE TO SUFFERING?

For most of us, the thought of death produces immediate fear, sadness, even despair. Yet death does not always equal suffering. For human beings who are themselves in the throes of terminal disease, death is a blessing. For family members, however, the fear of their loss frequently overcomes their ability to see this truth.

Over a long career in dealing with death and dying, I have found it necessary, on many occasions, to discuss this with distraught family members. I implore them to think not of their own pain, but of the best interest of their loved one. Frequently, this helps them make some of life's most difficult decisions—the discontinuation of life support, the decision not to continue aggressive, but futile, medical therapy.

Under the right circumstances, I point to the more spiritual aspects of death and dying, such as observations by survivors of the near-death experience, and the tremendous sense of peace and even great bliss that so many have reported.

Talking about death, in fact, can be the most liberating of experiences. What we try to suppress will only grow more powerful in our subconscious.

The Buddhists teach the impermanence of life very early on in the training of their young monks. Legend notes that the young initiates were required to sit and meditate among a number of dead bodies. This was not to depress them. It was meant to enlighten them. By accepting the reality of death as a basic truth they could move on to appreciate the value of life on a daily basis. It trained them to live each moment as the precious gift that it is, to understand that our physical bodies are programmed for a limited engagement here.

WHAT IS DEATH?

I am completely convinced that the death of the physical body does not mean the end of consciousness. To put it simply, the soul lives on. The awareness of this truth is a notion that can bring powerful healing to our lives. Acceptance of this notion can transform our fear of death and make our lives richer, fuller, and more productive.

Death is not the end. It is the transition to another state of being. The soul slips from the physical body back to the cosmos, to God, to the source of its being—whatever you prefer to call it. It alleviates the pain and suffering that often mark the inescapable decline and deterioration of this temporary vehicle we call the body. Death, for many, is the ultimate healing.

A NEW WAY TO EXPERIENCE DEATH AND LOSS

Death is not necessarily the tragedy it seems to be.

This notion may be too much to fathom when you are in the throes of grieving for a loved one who has died. We are mortal beings. Our emotions and feelings are the result of the love we shared with another, and we have every right to experience them fully when they occur. However, when you understand the true nature of death, it is possible to begin to see the death of a loved one as more than an enormous tragedy, more than the source of enormous personal pain and suffering.

If we can truly come to terms with this expanded notion of life, one independent of the physical body, it will be a tremendous source of healing from our grief.

For those experiencing the deterioration of their physical bodies, death can be regarded as a release and an unburdening of suffering. For those left behind, the process of mourning and moving on in life is a lesson for us as well.

We all suffer from the loss of those we love and who loved us. There will never be a way to avoid this inevitability. But we should also cultivate the awareness that our own suffering can be a selfish response to their leaving us behind. If we can see past our personal grief, we can be at peace with our loved one's liberation from a body that was ready to be discarded.

LOVE NEVER DIES

Our attachment to seeing and experiencing death as a tragic loss is the source of much of our fear and suffering. What if we came to believe that the essence of who we are is eternal? What if our most precious human feeling—love—did not dissolve into the universe when we or our loved ones died? What if we knew that our struggles in this lifetime were challenges our soul undertook prior to this incarnation?

There is no question that we would look at our own lives from a totally different perspective. We would never see ourselves as victims of the cruel winds of fate. We would find our losses and defeats more acceptable and be able to recover from them with less debilitating consequences.

By fearing death less, we could embrace life more. We could be more joyous and less depressed, and our energies could be applied to making this lifetime more meaningful.

We would finally understand that in order to be healthy and whole, we're required to have the awareness that we are body, mind, and spirit. We would know that loved ones never leave us and we never leave them, because love survives the end of the body. It lives in our hearts, and remains with the soul that goes on.

15

Suffering Is Not Punishment

I teach one thing and one thing only: suffering and the end of suffering.
—The Buddha

The Buddha, as well as all seekers of wisdom, struggled with the same basic questions of existence: How can we possibly reconcile the pain and suffering we see around us with a higher or deeper spiritual purpose?

Many schools of thought tell us that suffering is the inevitable consequence of "divine justice" acting on the inherent sinful nature of humanity. I, however, believe suffering represents the human mind's assessment of pain that is inherent in the physical world. This is the *distinction* between pain and suffering. Pain is universal; suffering varies considerably from one person to another. How we process this pain, and how we can use our awareness of the nature of reality to accept what we have no power to change, affects our degree of suffering.

This impermanent nature of all things is a universal truth. Buddhists in particular immerse themselves in this knowledge from an early age. This is not meant to depress the individual or impair their enjoyment in life. On the contrary, our typical Western approach—which is to deny the reality of death and to relegate the elderly and dying to hidden facilities—produces a deeper psychological disruption and cataclysm when the death of a loved one inevitably occurs. Suppression of emotions and fears only intensifies the power of our feelings.

To totally face and accept the inevitability of the death of all mortal beings allows us to move past this "beast with a thousand eyes" that seems to lurk below the surface of our consciousness like some mythological monster, ready to annihilate us. Face the fear and the monster shrinks before us in the light of awareness. Walk with the fear, and it loses its power to frighten us. It's very simple: to face this fear, and embrace life fully, *equals* less suffering.

Realization of the understanding that no one escapes this life without pain allows one to accept what comes our way with peace, equanimity, and understanding. Perhaps, if we realized that there are no free passes in this incarnation, that everyone—yes everyone—suffers, we would be less frustrated and angry over our own lives. We could finally escape the quicksand of envy and jealously. We could stop fantasizing about the lives of others, of trading places, as if only "they" have wonderful, beautiful lives. This delusion only serves to deny us what we so desperately seek: the ability to enjoy our own lives.

Perhaps if we understood that we should view life as managing imperfection, than we could stop making ourselves miserable. Some believe that our souls agree to certain contracts before birth, which will lead them into painful life situations. This would mean that pain is a natural part of the process of living.

Evil acts are a powerful cause of pain and suffering in this world, yet they do not argue necessarily against the existence of God or a higher spiritual reality. If we understand that our universe is based upon the notion of free will, then we must accept that God will/cannot interfere in the evil perpetrated by one human being against another. As uncomfortable as it may seem to us, God or the Supreme Intelligence could not stop Hitler, Stalin, Saddam Hussein, or any other brutal murderer from their freely chosen decisions.

In truth, unless our actions are totally free, acts of kindness and compassion would have no spiritual value either. So we must accept the nature of reality as it exists: free will allows for the horrors that we see around us. The redeeming factors, however, are this: (1) karma exists to address the evil actions and (2) our souls get many opportunities to return and do life over again. As I see it, each individual lifetime, as precious as it may be, is merely "survival weekend" in the context of infinity.

We must also see that tragedy opens the door to opportunities for the expression of loving kindness, compassion, and charity. These are truly spiritual gifts of grace.

For example, the sharing and self-sacrifice that occur after personal and natural disasters breaks through the barriers that we ordinarily erect to protect ourselves from intimacy and the fear of loss. When we touch the soul of another who is in pain, we heal that person and ourselves as well. Could it be the events that agitate pain and suffering are a natural part of life, designed to open our hearts and bring lessons of strength and courage in the face of calamity?

The human soul's desire to advance spiritually through free will acts of love and compassion would be rendered meaningless. To choose well—in a universe where evil is a real choice—allows us to heal ourselves and heal others.

Fear becomes a part of life the moment we attain human consciousness. We all have to face life's slings and arrows and we are frightened by this. Perhaps suffering is our gift. It challenges us to understand its nature, to accept its universality and to defy its propensity to suffocate us and to defeat us. It gives us the opportunity to choose good over evil, and love and compassion over fear and hate. Perhaps, in suffering, we find the ultimate meaning of existence for ourselves as healers.

16

Managing Our Imperfections

My imperfections and failures are as much a blessing from God as my successes and talents and I lay them both at His feet.
—Mahatma Gandhi

We are imperfect beings. We make mistakes, we hurt others, we undermine our own happiness and success, we lie to ourselves, we suffer. All of these qualities could turn us into miserable, despondent creatures. For some, the burden of living becomes overwhelming. For others, the lessons of despair bring spiritual riches and great wisdom.

The Buddha dedicated his life to the recognition and relief of suffering. His goal was to make people aware that suffering was natural to humanity, that we were here to learn through our challenges and losses, and that awareness of the cause of suffering could liberate us. Even the awareness of the universality of death was meant to enlighten us, not punish us.

There is a famous story from Buddhist legend about a young mother who was beyond consolation at the death of her young child. She ran around begging someone to help bring him back to life. An old wise woman suggested that she bring him to the Buddha. The Buddha saw the woman and child and said that he could bring the child back to life under one condition: That the woman collected a tamarind seed from every household who had not suffered a death in the family.

The woman proceeded to run from house to house begging for information about the lives of each family, desperate to come away with the seed. The truth was sadly apparent. No household had been spared the pain of death. She returned with her dead child to the Buddha without any seeds. He offered her his compassionate wisdom—life is impermanent and death must be recognized and accepted as a part of existence in this or any incarnation. According to legend, the woman was able to bury her son and went on to be a great Buddhist teacher.

There are no perfect lives "out there"—anywhere. It seems to be our human nature to dwell upon our individual suffering and to see others as having an easier time of it. Why do they have more ... live in bigger houses ... travel more ... seem happier than I do? The truth is that nobody escapes the inevitable—the general pain and suffering of existence. No one is free from physical, emotional, or mental stresses and strains. No one is completely happy, or completely sad. This is simply the way of the world, and it is actually okay.

We are all carrying around with us the wounds of past hurts—physical, emotional, or both. We are all the "walking wounded." The problem is not that we are imperfect. The problem is how we dwell on and label our imperfections. Rather than accepting them as part of life we tend to resist them or run from them.

It was not the Buddha's intention to torture that poor mother by having her make rounds of the homes of other people. He asked her to do so because he knew the realization of this truth could only come from her experience of it. One can be enlightened only through self-realization.

We can accept the pain yet reduce the suffering when we realize that this is the nature of all existence. As we come to understand that life is a series of tests, challenges, or obstacles for us to deal with and overcome, we begin to know firsthand that life, simply, is not perfect. Yet exploring its imperfection is the only way that we can test ourselves.

Imperfection is the nature of reality. Kabbalistic interpretations of the universe as shattered, and in need of repair, cast another light on imperfection. The world is imperfect, and this is so that we can help perfect it. Of course we can never truly achieve this goal. But just the awareness that we can try can raise our consciousness, our feelings of self-worth, and our compassion for fellow humans.

Another Kabbalistic teaching asks, "Where is God when people suffer?" The response is "God sends other people."

It is a profound teaching on several levels. It attempts to reassure us that there is a response to our suffering and that it is divinely inspired. It also demonstrates to us that we are each divine emissaries. We may not always be aware of this truth, but when we act with compassion and offer acts of loving kindness and charity, we are acting from a place of the divinity within ourselves.

History is replete with incidences in which individuals risked their own welfare and safety to assist other human beings. In recent times we have seen this in the aftermath of terrorist attacks, and natural disasters such as hurricanes, earthquakes and tsunamis. As ordinary citizens rise to the occasion of helping other human beings in need, we see glimpses of this higher spiritual consciousness as it manifests in the world.

Embracing our own difficulty allows us to help others through theirs. It offers us the opportunity to heal others while we heal ourselves.

17

Spiritually Correct Forgiveness

Our Father who art in Heaven.... Forgive us our trespasses as we forgive those who trespass against us.

—The Lord's Prayer

In almost any writings on spirituality there will be discussions of the unquestioned correctness of forgiveness. In short, forgiveness means letting go of negative feelings toward another who we feel has wronged us or someone we love.

It seems to be a favorite topic of Buddhist, Hindu, and Christian religious writing. Jewish and Islamic commentaries discuss this issue as well. There are books filled with quotes from each tradition extolling the virtues of forgiving one's enemy, regardless of the level of atrocities they may have committed.

Traditional Kabbalistic/Jewish teachings have emphasized that actions against another human being cannot be forgiven through prayer to God alone. However, direct admission of a wrongdoing to another person should be immediately followed by an acknowledgment of forgiveness. To withhold this statement based on a continual feeling of injustice or pain is to enter spiritually cloudy waters.

On a most pragmatic level, harboring resentments is like being imprisoned in a private hell. To hold tightly to negative feelings pollutes your own soul. In fact it binds you to someone whom you would prefer to be out of your life. An old Chinese proverb states that if you hold hatred in your heart for another, you might as well dig two graves. While you think you are "getting him back, alright!" it is you that suffers.

Requesting forgiveness from another whom we have wronged is by itself a spiritually enlightening act since it acknowledges that we may have hurt another living being. The act of seeking peace is always a *mitzvah*, a good deed. To mend and to bring harmony where there was a shattering of a relationship is a practical application of the Kabbalistic *tikkun* to repair or heal.

To do so is to promote peace in place of war, to establish order out of chaos. It is reminiscent of God's Biblical creation of the physical world. Such an action allows us to manifest our highest spiritual potential, as a cocreator with God.

As with any kind of healing—both parties benefit and both are healed by the process. It illustrates the Kabbalistic paradigm: heal your soul/heal the world. The two are mutually interconnected.

In all of our lives there are many times in which we hurt someone without the direct intention to do so—a careless comment, a joke that is taken as an offense, a sharp criticism of someone we truly love that arises out of our own hurt. All of these could be rationalized by any of us: "I didn't really mean any harm. I can't help it if they're too sensitive. I can't help it if they can't take a joke. That's their problem." Deep down we may feel justified in inflicting a bit of retribution.

These subtle forms of injury should be recognized as necessitating an action that leads to forgiveness and reconciliation. We need to be empathic with one another rather than defensive. Empathy is love, it is compassion. It breaks down barriers.

Each of us needs to be the one who makes the first step—toward love and away from hurt. Each one of us must forgive first, not wait for the other to do so. An act of privately seeking to soothe the injured ego of another is the highest of spiritual deeds.

We often live our lives inside protective shells. We fear being hurt so much that we don't connect with others at all. Our defensive barriers are so strong that they block all feeling, to any connection with another. In this scenario, we anesthetize ourselves to emotion. We become frozen.

The act of approaching another who feels we have wronged them can be like picking up an ice pick. At first, it may appear to be another attack, but make that first chip and the ice will begin to crumble. Long-suppressed pent-up emotions can be released. In this act of compassion, true healing can occur. It may require an enormous act of our free will to make that first move. We worry that our approach may be rebuffed. We know that we are putting ourselves in a place where we could be hurting even more. But to do so is an incredible act of spiritual courage.

There are many people in our lives with whom we share an ambivalent relationship. Usually these individuals have hurt us; but it is often unconsciously, out of a sense of their own inadequacies, and from a place of their own pain. The ability to see that truth, to feel compassion for another who has hurt us, is the basis upon which we can forgive them.

A good friend of mine had spoken to me about his childhood, how he was always put down by his father as someone who would never be a success in life. He harbored a great deal of anger and resentment toward his father and actually became an amazing father for his own sons. Over the past few years, however, as his own spiritual awareness grew, he begun to see his father in a different light. He realized that his father had grown up with his own deep pain and insecurities, that his father did love him but was just unable to give more to him than he did. He recently thanked his father for showing him how *not to be* a parent. (He was not being bitter or facetious.) He told him that he understood that he did the best that he could, that he loved him and forgave him. Talk about healing! When we forgive it means we own up to our responsibility in the forgiveness game.

But what about the forgiving when it involves unprovoked violence toward those we love or the country we love? In the absence of the perpetrator's acknowledgment or participation, forgiveness offers particular spiritual challenges. There is no shortage of horrific acts that seem completely unforgivable—murders, genocides, atrocities of war, suicide bombers, September 11 . . . the list goes on.

Desire for retribution, revenge, and a cry for justice may be immediate reactions to these activities. But when the search for fairness, to right something, leads to further acts of hatred, can it ever be a winning situation?

Does the word *forgiveness* have any meaning under these dire circumstances? Can we even find it in our hearts and minds to consider? Could we ask that of those who have lost someone close, someone loved? It certainly tests our souls.

To forgive does not mean to forget. To forgive does not mean to *excuse the behavior* of others. Forgiveness does not invalidate self-defense or even preemptive attacks against an inevitable foe. But to defend oneself does not necessitate dehumanizing another human being. It does not mean reveling in their defeat. However despicable and debased their actions, they are humans whose suffering has blinded them to the true nature of their actions.

Buddhists speak of defending themselves, even disarming a perpetrator but not harboring feelings of hatred for that individual. Compassion is extended to all beings even those who threaten to harm others. It is understood that those that commit acts of violence are not at peace themselves. Hatred is a powerfully dark emotion that corrupts anyone who harbors it.

I have always been deeply moved by one particular Passover ritual. It occurs during the Seder when the Ten Plagues are enumerated. These represent the incremental punishing of the Pharaoh and the Egyptians in their refusal to release the Israelite slaves.

A drop of wine is removed from the glass of the participants in the Seder for each plague enumerated in order to show compassion for the suffering of those same Egyptians who held the Israelites in bondage. *The Haggadah*, the traditional guidebook used for Passover seders, clearly states that one is not to rejoice in the suffering of others. It is a symbolic act of forgiveness that empowers those who participate in this ritual.

To forgive does not mean to *accept the actions* of others as justified. To forgive means to release ourselves from the prison of hatred and free our hearts of its burden.

Maybe we need a new word for forgiveness? Or a new way of looking at the seemingly unforgivable. Perhaps trust in a higher form of cosmic justice is helpful. Many spiritual traditions look to karma, or its equivalent, to explain the inequality and imbalance that seems to exist all around us. They proclaim the belief that order will be restored, and it is not up to us, personally, to do it.

Forgiveness calls upon us to transcend our usual human reactivity, our defensiveness, our fear. It asks of us to rise above our habitual behavior. It pleads with us to understand and have compassion for another human being who struggles with the challenges of existence as we do. It requires us to seek our Higher Self, the part of us that is Divine, and to remember that we are here to learn and to grow spiritually. Forgiveness challenges us to do just that.

18

Kavanah: The Intention to Do Good

Our intention creates our reality.

—Wayne Dyer

In the fast pace of modern life, it is not so easy to tap into our purest desires. Nor is it easy to do for others just for the sake of doing, or give of ourselves because it is what we are meant to do here on earth.

In everyday life, we spend so much time doing things to impress others or to make ourselves look good. We do things to advance our careers and our agendas. We do things because we must, because our families, clients, or bosses demand it.

Can we be truly motivated by the spirit of the joy of giving, not the attitude of duty or sacrifice?

The Kabbalistic notion of *kavanah* means *intention* or *desire*. It is associated with the inner feeling, or motivation, to do something, to achieve a goal, to connect with our Higher Self.

From a Kabbalistic perspective, intention is as important as deed. The traditional activity associated with *kavanah* is prayer. Anyone can go through the motions and read the words, while actually letting the mind wander, or getting distracted, thinking about where to go for dinner, or wondering about the attractive woman in the next aisle. That we often forget our focus at the precise performance of ritual or prayer itself is what makes it sacred—and effective. Rabbis emphasize that performing a good deed, a mitzvah, without *kavanah*, is to fail to tap into the spiritual energy of the action.

There is a fascinating Kabbalistic story about a small synagogue in Eastern Europe in the days before Hitler. On one of the High Holidays, Yom Kippur, the most solemn day of the year for observant Jews, all the men were praying in their usual fashion, saying the words, speaking to each other, looking around. A young boy who had just begun to study the Hebrew alphabet began to shout out the letters, one after the other. It was obvious to all that he had not yet learned the prayers.

The boy's father tried to keep him quiet, "shushing" him as he continued to yell the alphabet as loudly as he could. The elderly rabbi, seeing the commotion, did something totally unheard of—he stopped the services. Everyone became quite alarmed. They had never seen anything like it. The rabbi climbed off the bimah (the altar/stage) and walked straight to the boy and his father. The father was literally sweating and shaking, as this rabbi was held in such esteem.

Appearing like a biblical prophet, the holy man with a flowing white beard and dressed in total white talis and robes looked at both of them and said, "How dare you try to quiet this young boy? He may not know the words but because he prays from such *kavanah*, the heavens are open for all of your prayers!"

It demonstrates that our intention to do good—to perform acts of kindness, to offer charity when someone asks for it, or to offer healing—is a spiritual power not only to those who receive but to those who give. And it reminds us that this purity of motivation dwells within us all.

On a mystical level, *kavanah* does something else, something quite fascinating. By intending to do something, we stop the flow of time. By our intention to perform an action with compassion or kindness, we set off ripples of loving energy that span the universe at the speed of a thought. The Universe listens. It is telling us that what we think counts as much as what we do.

Part VI
Choosing Healing as a Way of Life

Hasidism popularized Kabbalah's notion that all of life is in need of healing and fixing, not just those who are ill. It affirmed the Kabbalah's deeply optimistic view that however broken and fragmented things may seem, all life is in fact evolving toward a state of wholeness. . . . Each of us, taught the Hasidic masters, has the power to become a holy fixer and healer.

—Estelle Frankel

19

Healing—What Does It Really Mean?

Healing is not the same as curing, after all; healing does not mean going back to the way things were before, but allowing what is now to move closer to God.

—Ram Dass

I use the term *healing* in ways that may challenge some traditional notions.

To heal means to "make whole," to achieve a level of completeness, of fulfillment. And who among us is not whole? All of us! When it comes to our minds, our thoughts and emotions are often fragmented and confused, embroiled in a continuous struggle to make sense of our lives. As regards to our body, our immune system is never at rest, constantly battling invading bacteria, viruses, and carcinogens.

Healing is not a state of being, but a process of becoming whole. We are usually unaware of it, since it occurs subconsciously and internally. It is silent and protective. We know about it only when it fails.

Our minds strain against the strangle hold of anxiety, sadness, loneliness, fear of failure, the fear of success, and the fear of fear. Healing is always a dynamic process, always in motion. It never rests.

The emphasis on the term *process* is important. None of us ever truly reach complete and perfect health, and even the most well put together of us are never completely whole in mind, body, and spirit. Our bodies, for example, wage a losing battle to repair and restore the vigor of our middle years. The ability of our cells to perform such tasks wanes as the setting sun. *Senescence* is the term for this gradual failure to maintain the status quo—it is the name of the process that leads to our inevitable physical demise.

True, a human being is an amazingly complex and capable self-healing organism. Assistance from others, however, is often required in this process. We may regard ourselves as an "island universe," but in fact we are social beings who cannot live without each other.

The act of healing, or attempting to heal another, begins with recognition of the state of isolation that all beings inherently experience. This is the source of our primal state of fear. Healing on this deep level represents the triumph of love over fear, as manifested by acts of compassion, of caring. It has powerfully spiritual ramifications for both healer and healee. To be in need of healing is human, to attempt to heal others is an act of compassion and empathy that reflects the part of us that is divine.

In Kabbalistic terms, the world is broken, shattered. Human beings are endowed through acts of free will with the capacity to assist in the act of *tikkun* or repair. This healing is the purpose of our existence on this physical plane. It allows our soul to grow and develop on a personal as well as cosmic level.

Buddhism recognizes that all human beings suffer. This suffering is a consequence of our ignorance about the nature of reality and the reasons behind our suffering. To overcome this suffering through acts of awareness, compassion, kindness, and caring are healing to our Higher Self. We accrue karmic credits through healing our suffering and the suffering of those around us.

Christian salvation requires acts of faith rather than deeds. It frees the troubled soul, an act of healing as well. In fact spiritual transformation of any kind, from nearly any tradition, establishes the purpose of existence: it is not only to serve God but to become more God-like. Our human failings are the evidence that we are in need of healing. Our embracing of a higher morality based upon the Golden Rule of "do unto others as we would have do unto us" is the source of our spiritual energy.

Disease states are often regarded by the medical establishment as a consequence of one or more of the three *bad*'s: bad genes, bad behavior, and bad luck.

Everyone is aware, for example, that genes play a role in the tendencies to develop certain diseases. Behavior plays an enormous role as well. Smoking, eating unhealthy foods, excessive alcohol, drugs, and chronic emotional disturbances all have a well-known impact on the body's immune response: to resist infectious agents and derail malignancies early in their development. And what about chance? Here we are entering the realm of uncertainty. Does illness strike without warning? Do our souls conspire, prior to this incarnation, to face challenges to our mind and body?

There are many tools on this path toward healing and all can be called upon when they are needed. Western scientific accomplishments—in terms of pharmaceutical advances and technological accomplishment—can clearly aid in the treatment of the physical body. We should welcome them as the products of the human mind, and therefore the results of the evolutionary process itself. There are some supporters of alternative therapies who regard traditional medicine as restrictive and controlling. They may automatically reject it as the product of big drug companies and organized medicine. There are many individuals who will embrace any alternative therapy without carefully examining and analyzing its effectiveness and safety profile. They are in danger of falling into the trap that "natural" therapies are automatically safer and better.

The most sensible approach, I believe, is to retain an open-minded skepticism as it regards *all* therapies, traditional and alternative. Evaluate the evidence in well-done studies to see which therapies work and which do not. Evaluate the risk of the therapy and potential side effects versus the benefits. No therapy, no pill, and no herbal preparation is without potential toxicity. So be aware and be vigilant. But don't avoid therapies that may be helpful because of excessive fear of potential side effects.

I do not believe that traditional and alternative therapies are mutually exclusive whatsoever. In fact, the term that seems most appropriate today is CAM (complementary and alternative medicine). The open hand of compassion combined with the technological advancements of contemporary technology offer us our best hope for healing. Technology alone cannot address issues of mind and soul, which are crucial to the process of healing. Technology does not "heal." Its true role is to "assist" the natural processes, which are in continuous motion.

Healing means becoming more at peace with the emotional and physical battles that rage within us. The Taoist notion of Yin and Yang acknowledges the balanced flow between opposites that characterizes the nature of reality. The notion of balance, peace, and joy are important in the process of healing. Happiness and sadness, rest and activity, eating in moderation—all acknowledge that a balance in everything produces a state of healing.

Healing requires the courage to face our own responsibility in this process. We cannot turn our bodies over to a physician and expect to be "fixed" as one would a car. We are required to do "work," to be present and to seek acceptance of what our physical body decides to do.

Healing means evolving. Healing means learning about ourselves and the world around us. Healing means facing our challenges with determination and confidence. Healing means learning to face our darkest fears, our deepest sources of grief and despair, and to choose to find meaning in those most difficult moments. Healing is about managing the imperfection that is life with the courage that we will prevail.

20

Healing through Gratitude

I wake up each morning and say, it's a miracle! I'm alive!
—Rabbi Joseph Gelberman, Ph.D.

Many of us are dissatisfied with our lives—many are frustrated, bored, depressed, and anxious. We are discontent, unhappy—but what are we all looking for? We live in a society and culture that offers us easy access to material goods. We appreciate very little because we live in a world of such abundance. We are told that our cars are not good enough, our spouses are not sexy enough, our clothes are behind the times, our homes are inadequate, our careers mediocre, and our looks are less than magnificent.

At times we are exposed to overwhelming pictures of poverty, usually on TV news and heart-wrenching commercials. We turn our heads from such sadness and degradation. We notice how precious even simple toys, clothes, and a morsel of food are to such children and we are rightfully embarrassed by our own abundance.

Still, we are grateful for very little. Instead, we want more. We demand more and believe that what will satisfy us is more of what we already have. It is never about the intangibles: love, relationships, families, friends, health, contentment, a sense of peace. We have all forgotten one of life's most obvious lessons—cultivating a state of mind in which gratitude is present is ultimately healing. It can offer us much of what we are seeking: a sense of peace and contentment.

Money, career, properties, vacations, net worth, cars, the colleges, and even our children's careers: enumerating a list of our wants becomes our list of demands on life. If other people can have them, then why can't we obtain them as well? We are competitive. Life seems to be a contest in which the winner has more of everything than anyone else. Yet this aggressive aspect rarely brings a sense of wholeness or contentment. How can it?

We are so driven by the process of acquiring that we can barely enjoy what we do have. Even love and friendship is seen as a commodity. How many dear friends do you have, or, more important, how many successful, well-regarded, or famous people do you count among your friends? How many calls or e-mails do you receive that are not spam or telemarketers? How many invitations do you receive to social events?

We have all but forgotten the simple, satisfying beauty of gratitude. It is a way of acknowledging the wonder of existence. Cultivating a mind of gratitude forces us to look at what we value in our lives and step outside of our cultural and societal patterns.

Several years ago, I noticed that I would become emotionally drained by the many patients I saw in my office on any given day. At times I would resent their demands or attitudes, or the fees that insurance companies would pay me for my time and effort. I wasn't having much fun or enjoyment either. Then I learned about the Kabbalistic lesson that beggars in Jerusalem understood. They knew that their presence, their outstretched hand would offer another individual an opportunity to perform a mitzvah, an act of charity that brought spiritual benefits to them. I began to see that the patients who entered my examination room were offering me an opportunity to do good deeds or *mitzvot*. I became grateful for their presence and my energy levels swelled concomitantly. No longer drained by the patient–doctor encounter, I actually was energized by virtue of my gratitude.

Small acts of gratitude go a long way. Feeling grateful for the morning, for an opportunity to live another day, for a smile, for a chance to help someone with an act of kindness—these are all empowering to both giver and recipient. Just telling your loved ones you are grateful for having them in your life is an act of love and thoughtfulness that is soothing and healing to you both. It costs nothing yet it is priceless. And it leads to contentment and joy.

Gratitude requires us to freeze the frenetic pace of life—to stop in our tracks and to live in the moment—because only if we stop time can we acknowledge that we appreciate anything. Gratitude requires that we explore the good and fulfilling aspects of our life and allow the negative and painful elements to stand back for a while. Clearly, we have not forgotten that we live imperfect lives. In fact, we usually are *so* focused on what is missing, what is incomplete—our losses and frustrations—that we spoil what is truly amazing about our lives.

Gratitude takes us out of our own sadness for a moment. It shakes us out of our victim mentality and breaks our egocentric perspective on life. It moves us to be appreciative of something or someone outside of ourselves. It shows us that we are connected to others, and helps us see ourselves within a larger context.

Gratitude allows us to find a spiritual sense of ourselves, to be grateful for being alive, no matter how bad our lives seem.

Holocaust survivor and psychiatrist Viktor Frankl, author of *Man's Search for Reason*, has correlated survival in concentration camps with an individual's ability to find meaning in the smallest piece of existence. Even the sight of a new bud on a spring branch became a joyous reason to keep living. With such gratitude for life, people are able to survive life's most unbearable moments with a sense of hope.

Gratitude allows us to see life's difficulties as temporary setbacks and it shields us from despair, self-depreciation, and getting lost in life's little—and big—detours from success and wellness.

Being grateful may not come naturally to many of us. It may require that we exercise our free will and choose how we perceive and experience life. It may move us to train our minds, to stop ourselves from falling into old patterns of negative thinking and reacting. Sometimes, at our lowest points, we have to remind ourselves to be grateful for what we have. And for what we've had.

In any crisis, an attitude of gratitude can help you get through the dark days. It is an enormous healing when you learn to live with a sense of true gratitude.

21

Healing through Happiness

I believe that the very purpose of our life is to seek happiness.

—The Dalai Lama

Joy is a rare but precious feeling. At times it arises predictably from positive life events: the birth of a child, the advancement in one's chosen career, an expression of love from a fellow human being. Joy can arise from an experience of nature, a sudden inspiration that conveys a new understanding of our place in the universe.

Joy can also, at times, appear from nowhere. Unbidden, and unexpected, this is the most incredible perception of all. I refer to this experience as a "spontaneous feeling of joy," or SPJ. It may very well be a gift from our soul. It is often short-lived and we may soon forget that it even occurred. For we are soon back in our usual state of consciousness—battling the demons of work, time, expectations, disappointments, and frustrations.

I would propose that we regard these SPJ as spiritual bonus—energy boosters, if you will, to keep us going through the difficult times in our lives. I also believe that we can magnify them, even store them in our memories, keeping them available for retrieval when we most need them. We need not question them—merely nurture them.

The Dalai Lama describes happiness as man's most basic drive. The source of our own happiness occurs when we forget about ourselves—literally when our own egos disappear from view—and we are present with another human being sharing our compassionate concern for him or her.

It is precisely when we *don't* anticipate our own happiness that we experience it.

An elderly patient recently appeared in my office with gastrointestinal complaints that she could ascribe to stress. At first, the source of that stress seemed to be involved with her elderly, ill husband. Soon, however, she said, "I don't think I mentioned this to you, but my son committed suicide about a year ago."

Her next words were powerfully revealing, "Don't let anyone tell you that money buys happiness. He was an enormously successful attorney and businessman. His personal life, however, was in shambles. He had been divorced and had poor relations with his adult children. His second marriage was crumbling, and he had developed medical problems as well. I had no idea that he was so depressed. What was even more devastating was his last note, in which he stated he had no reason to live. No reason? Didn't he think about me, his mother?"

While lack of money can be a source of suffering, it is our personal relationships, our feeling of being loved in spite of our frailties, that give us the sustenance to go on, to heal.

One of the hallmarks of happiness is it allows us to regard life's trickier moments as opportunities for learning. It may hurt to lose a job, be rejected by a lover, or experience a failure or loss that makes us feel we are heading in the wrong direction. Yet when we come at this from a generally happy attitude about life, we can override the tendency to lose confidence and sink into despair. Although the going can get tough when it feels like the rug has been pulled out from under, we have to sometimes fight to remind ourselves it is not the end of the world.

From the perspective of outsiders looking in, it may seem that your world has fallen apart because, frankly, many people tend to view loss as extremely negative and demoralizing—a tragedy. And even if you seem to be "okay with it," there will be plenty of people who will think you are in denial.

There are a plethora of ways and means by which the average person creates his or her own sense of reality from among the fragments of his or her life. The truth is, if you choose to see your loss as a transformation and opportunity to change, you will, eventually, transform your reality into opportunities rather than feeling like a loser.

Even a major change can be regarded as a temporary roadblock and you can use the time of transition to become more skillful, redirect yourself on your chosen path or choose a different one, or to simply alter your life's journey and set sail for new horizons.

If you take the higher road, you will be filled with energy and hope for the future. Even though a similar set of circumstances could totally depress and demoralize people around you, and give them a sob story they can use forever, you can choose happiness, and new ways of experiencing it!

Tailoring our reaction to life's events is something many of us would like to master. Words and phrases are powerful signals to our conscious as well as unconscious minds. Seeing ourselves as failures, victims, or losers in life's game merely reinforces and exacerbates the negative energy that can only cripple us further. It is unproductive!

It should be obvious that a joyous, positive self-awareness will be far more effective in healing than the opposite. Joy is a positive stimulant of our body's inherent healing properties. We will likewise attract more enriching human emotional responses from others as well.

Perhaps the most reasonable approach to life is this: seek the highest level of optimism that allows us to heal our wounds. Choose happiness whenever possible since this is clearly the state of being that fills our hearts and minds with healing energy. Be aware of our chosen path and if there is a persistent lack of progress toward our self-proclaimed goals, be willing to modify and revisit those goals. Altering or redirecting our energies does not have to be seen as failure.

22

Healing through Sadness

The Lord is close to the brokenhearted and saves those who are crushed in spirit.

—Psalm 34:18

Sadness seems to defy the very notion of healing. Rather, all spiritual traditions point to a state of joy as essential to approach the Divine.

Enlightenment is always pictured as a smiling Buddha, an ecstatic saint. Kabbalistic and Hindu writings share similar notions that one should not leave one's abode without a smile. To do so is to impose your negative energy on others as well as to doubt the ultimate goodness of the creation. The Baal Shem Tov, founder of Hasidism, noted that the transmission of joy through the act of smiling is such a profound spiritual act as to justify one's entire incarnation in this lifetime.

Healing means to make whole, and sadness seems to render one fragmented and frustrated. Sadness seems to weaken us, as if someone has tapped our vital energy and allowed it to dissipate. But there is an element to sadness that is essential to life itself. We are not automatons; we feel the ordinary ups and downs that are inherent in this life. We will all be disappointed, upset, and rejected. We will not have everything go as planned. We will certainly not win every contest in life. We will ultimately lose those we love and cherish. We will hurt. It may not be fun, but, most important, we would never appreciate joy without its counterpart, sadness.

Sadness can carry important lessons for us. It is the consequence of emotional pain. And just as physical pain is necessary to alert us that our body needs immediate attention, sadness serves the same function for our emotional self. In addition to normal feelings of mourning, loss, the blues, sadness can also tell us when we need to make some changes in our lives. Sadness can be an early alert about a bigger problem, such as depression that needs to be treated, or it can be a passing phase based on what is going on in our lives.

Our understanding of sadness is complicated by our cultural perspective on it. We live in a culture that seeks to escape sadness as soon as it arises.

To deal with the underlying causes is a far different approach than to seek an immediate fix. We are a "pill-taking" society and will often seek an immediate relief of our symptoms. Pharmaceutical companies and physicians contribute to the belief that we should anesthetize ourselves to any negative feelings. The amount of antianxiety and antidepressant drugs prescribed in this country is astounding. This may contribute to an attitude of feeling better without addressing the underlying causes of sadness and ultimately depression. Troubled personal and professional lives are not addressed directly. Instead, these serious issues are buried by mood-elevating drugs and use of alcohol. Healing can never take place under these circumstances. Because sadness offers an enormous challenge to our sense of self, it forces us to explore our inner fears and to seek to repair them. Whereas sadness is a normal part of life, when unrecognized through denial or suppression it can progress into depression, which is more difficult to treat. This is why healing through sadness is such a powerful notion.

It is easy to smile when the sun is shining, all our plans seem blessed, things are going our way and we feel loved and protected. When we fear failure, disappointment, loneliness we pull back into a shell. Of course, the irony is that this act only further isolates us from the love of others as well as the self-love that can liberate us from sadness and fear. What greater challenge is there than to find light hidden under darkness?

Kabbalistic metaphors offer considerable insight to the topic of sadness. We speak of being fragmented or broken by life's challenges, which frequently lead to sadness. Ironically, Kabbalistic images of the creation of the world describe the shattering of primal vessels. Such a catastrophe at the beginning of creation would seem to lead to the ultimate destruction and a premature demise of the physical universe. The sparks of divinity are scattered throughout the physical world and become trapped in shells, *kelipot*. The strong implication is that the world contains a spark of divinity, a soul, regardless of whether it is inanimate or animate. Humankind's role in creation, therefore, is to liberate these holy sparks through acts of kindness, compassion, charity, and humility and by following the commandments.

This is *tikkun*, the repair and healing of the universe. This requires an active role for mankind in cocreating the world. It rejects passivity and depression by insisting that humanity assume its role. This could not have been achieved without sadness. Unless the universe becomes broken, and humanity fulfills its highest destiny, we cannot participate in the healing of the world.

When sadness outlives its usefulness and drifts into depression, then breaking free becomes a necessary act of choice, of pure will. To do so may seem to some as an act of delusion, or irrational "spinning" of one's life's events. Yet the ultimate purpose is to recast reality in a manner that will allow us to break out of these chains of despair and to heal. Spiritual thinkers have always acknowledged that the greatest achievement is to achieve holiness from the depths of darkness. Overcoming sadness recognizes this transformation. It is the ultimate form of healing.

23

Age of Addiction

> Every form of addiction is bad no matter whether the narcotic is alcohol or morphine or idealism.
>
> —Carl Jung

For those who consider themselves free of addictions . . . don't be so sure. *Addiction* is just another term for "habitual behavior that we adopt in order to relieve anxiety and frustration."

Anything we do can be or become addictive if approached without mindfulness and awareness. This includes being addicted to substances, material things, people, experiences, feelings, and anything else that we may use to take ourselves from ordinary reality, and which reduces anxiety, dampens fear, and temporarily gives us a high.

Like most forms of human behavior, what distinguishes pathological behavior—from a "variation" of normal—is a matter of degree and interpretation.

Evolutionary biology is a fairly recent field of science that essentially acknowledges that much of human behavior exists because of some evolutionary benefit to our species. The ability to soothe our anxieties and fears is an example of this adaptive behavior. Pathological states become evident, however, when these "normal" adaptive behaviors, or mechanisms for survival, cross the line. When they involve the use of illegal substances, or become obsessive in their use, that is when we are no longer using them but they are using us.

Some of us pray, others do yoga and meditate, some exercise vigorously, and others utilize combinations of all of the above. Some seek professional help with therapy and prescription drugs. When the methods we seek to help us get through life are considered excessive, when they seem to control us rather than we control them, they are labeled as addictions.

Our culture deems certain addictions more dangerous, damaging or unacceptable than others. Drugs and alcohol are looked upon as killers of people and life itself. Addicts literally kill themselves with their drug of choice. Smoking is seen as the horrible habit that makes everyone sick—the smoker and those exposed to it. Gambling is another addiction that brings down individuals and those around them. Video games and the Internet—not to mention the usual suspects, food, sex, and shopping—can lead to excessive problem behaviors in our modern age.

Addictive behavior is often viewed as the path of the emotionally and intel-lectually weak. But is that really true? Some of us are smart, high-functioning addicts who quietly do our thing and keep coming back for more, with no one being the wiser about our behavior. It doesn't fit into a classic "addiction" model so maybe no one really notices. How can you tell you are addicted? Anytime you have to "have, be, do" something, you are hooked.

What begins as something that takes the edge off emotional and physical pain, or gives you a little crutch to lean on when going through a tough time, becomes something you feel you cannot be without. Some of us take this "relief" too far, and make it dangerous for ourselves and others. We get so deep into it that a physical need kicks in and makes it harder and harder to control. Certain chemicals are known to be particularly "addictive," creating extremely uncomfortable symptoms when an individual tries to withdraw (such as nicotine) or requiring medical intervention (such as opiates, amphetamines, and cocaine). Sometimes we stay with our addictions because they are simply too hard to leave, and we have so little tolerance for the "detox."

It doesn't matter how smart you are, or even how strong your will is in some cases. Addiction takes on a life of its own. Most substance abusers are physically unable to just walk away without experiencing significant physical distress. Ad-dictions tend to be a mixture of physical and emotional dependency. This is why the emotional and spiritual aspect of overcoming addiction—of any kind—is so important.

Many people are cross-addicted, or try to replace one addiction with another. If it is our habit to reach for food, drugs, alcohol, or a sexual experience to substitute a bad feeling for a good feeling, then there is a tendency to reach for "something" even when we are in recovery from another addiction. For example, a food addict might take up shopping, instead of eating, or could get so completely devoted to exercise that exercise is the new extreme. For the moment, they can lose themselves in the pleasurable experience—spending money or spending calories.

Some people just become chronic volunteers who can't stop doing things for others, and some become activity addicts, whether it be trolling garage sales every Saturday or going to sports functions or theater. Whatever the addiction, there is a temporary high that makes people keep coming back.

There is little doubt that human beings are susceptible to being swept up by the rhetoric and ideologies of large movements. History is replete with such examples and most, unfortunately, have led to wars, pogroms, and other atrocities. The ability of individuals to "lose themselves" to the doctrines and dogmas groups is a form of addiction.

One of the most powerful lessons that can be learned by opening oneself up to personal metaphysical inquiry is this: think for oneself. Question everything, especially the emotionally charged claims of leaders who find scapegoats to blame for everything.

Religious and political movements, cults, gangs, and movements that submerge our individuality into a "group-think" can alleviate our individual anxieties and concerns. We can become emotionally and psychologically addicted because we find comfort and relief from our own problems when we follow the group's dictates. In this we see extremes too, from groups (some called cults) of people maintaining an addiction to a leader or a cause.

Addictions tend to focus us in the present with little regard for future ramifications. It is all about now. It is all about feeling good, now! Ironically, this may be one example in which "living in the moment" is not helpful whatsoever. It is truly an escape from the future, of consequences, of facing being discovered, of having to come to terms with that which is being avoided.

The lesson for healing is clear. Avoidance, repression of painful feelings, is not the path to wholeness. Chemical ingestions of drugs allow us to postpone confronting the realities of our own lives. Even carbohydrates or shopping online can give us a temporary surge of dopamine, endorphins, and serotonin that carries us away from worries—in that moment. Acceptance of these painful experiences "face on" is extremely difficult, and traumatic, yet we can help meet them head on with awareness and mindfulness. Eventually, we can become skillful at a way of approaching life that is not addictive, or self-destructive.

The path of mindfulness meditation offers a healing alternative. This technique centers on an awareness of the breath, the flow in and out, while allowing thoughts and emotions to flow in and out of our attention. We remain "present" and aware of these thoughts and feelings but do not "attach" to them.

We assume a position as witness to everything that enters our consciousness. By not denying or repressing them, they lose their power over us, our need to escape them through potentially addictive behavior. By witnessing them, we can stand aside and not be overwhelmed by them. It is a healing modality that we could all benefit from.

By reaching deep within, we can touch the spiritual core of our being and become aware of the reason for our being here: to face challenges to our mind and body and to overcome them.

Slipping into addictive behaviors is like playing hooky from the school of life. We are here to learn and grow, not hide and cop out. The best way to go through the classroom of life is by staying present and participating fully. We may be tempted to cut school or tune out from time to time, but those who stick it out can graduate and move on to new phases of life—rather than get stuck in the rut of addiction.

24

The Placebo Effect: Proof of the Body–Mind Connection?

One should treat as many patients as possible with a new drug while it still has the power to heal.

—Sir William Osler, Father of Modern Medicine

"Believe it . . . or not." You have heard that statement many times in your life, followed usually by another statement to be pondered. But stop with the first phrase—there is wisdom in it. What you believe to be true will kill you . . . or cure you.

That, in essence, is the lesson of the placebo effect. Some time in the first few months of my medical school rotation in internal medicine, I was exposed to the concept of the placebo. It was described by my senior residents as an inactive sugar pill, or an injection of saline. If a patient was in pain and responded with the relief of their pain after a placebo, the conclusion was clear—the patient was "faking" his or her symptoms. Somehow, we were taught, they were never in pain, otherwise how could their pain be relieved by the inactive placebo?

As an impressionable medical student all those many years ago I too bought into the notion that the placebo effect was evidence for an unreliable, deceitful, and untrustworthy patient. Now, I cringe at that thought. Did I actually project those feelings to those unfortunate patients?

And now the truth is clear—those patients were in pain, and they did perceive what they claimed to feel. The benefit of the placebo was demonstrating something so profound and real that we—the medical establishment—were unable and unwilling to comprehend it. The mind and the body are so inextricably linked that the belief that something will work will actually activate biochemical mechanisms within the body–brain that will accomplish what the drug was intended to do.

Science has finally found the evidence of a truth that has been known by spiritual traditions for millennia—that our minds and higher consciousness can influence our physical being. Of course the reverse is certainly true as well—the events in our lives, interpreted by our minds as positive or negative, will have a profound impact upon our body's defenses.

Research into the field of psychoneuroimmunology (PNI) has offered science the proof of this connection, something that many scientists had long denied. It also explained something else quite profound—our bodies have evolved with the ability to calm ourselves, sedate ourselves, relieve anxiety and depression, and to provide pain relief and even deep sleep.

This awareness became clear to me in my own practice while performing thousands of endoscopic procedures on patients under anesthesia. In order for any anesthetic agent to have a sedating effect upon the patient, it had to bind to pre-existing receptors in the brain. These sites evolved over millions of years, clearly before the discovery of anesthetics or other mind-altering drugs for a reason. That reason is simple: our ancestors, those whose brains contained receptors to essentially "heal" their emotional disturbances, survived to pass along this capability to us.

We are biologically programmed to heal our own anxiety, depression, or insomnia. This is a rather astounding observation and one that should inspire us all to seek to develop our own capacity to tap into this truth—to heal ourselves.

Pharmaceutical companies learned to create artificial compounds that would bind with these natural receptors sites. They did not invent these sites—they simply discovered how to activate them. If we could learn how to tap into our own production of these peptides, we could put the drug companies out of business. The example of the placebo effect should embolden us to do it!

The good news is that there are a variety of ways in which an individual can tap into their own mood-altering, receptor-binding peptides. The classic example, known to many, is that of endorphins, natural opiates, that are released by a variety of human activities, including exercise, sexual activity, meditation, prayer, hypnosis, and other self-induced behaviors.

The fact that placebos have the power to produce effects in subjects taking them has provided the pharmaceutical companies with tremendous headaches. They must demonstrate to the FDA that their drug—which may have cost a billion dollars to research and develop—will outperform an inexpensive inert placebo. This is not easily done. Studies have shown that placebos induce improvement in symptoms in anywhere from 35 to 50 percent of patients studied!

Issues involving the ability of our bodies to fight infections and cancer are also clearly relevant to the mind–body connection. While acute jolts of stress actually enable our bodies to quickly assume a posture to either fight or escape as well as to defend against infectious agents, chronic persistent stress places an enormous burden on our defense mechanisms—rendering them incapable of defending against infections and cancer.

Our state of mind is what counts where our immune system is concerned. The *nocebo* effect is the mirror image of the placebo response. Anticipating adverse effects from an inert, inactive pill results in unfavorable reactions to it. Once again, what we believe will happen, will happen. How we think, feel, believe about ourselves and about how our bodies will react actually make it so.

Our culture relies too heavily on treating disease and ailments via drugs, surgery, and procedures. The placebo effect tells us that taking responsibility for our own healing is not such a far-fetched idea and that we should at least investigate the power of our minds to change the responses in our physical being.

25

Obesity and How to Avoid It: A Weighty Metaphysical Topic

> There are two primary choices in life: to accept conditions as they exist or accept the responsibility for changing them.
> —Dennis Waitley

Food. We can't live without it—literally. Eating is so basic to our daily lives that it can become either a dumping ground for our emotional conflicts and agonies or an opportunity to be mindful of our lives several times a day.

We are a society obsessed with obesity and how to avoid it. This is a relatively modern issue for humanity. For most of our evolution, and still in large parts of the third world, starvation is a far greater and prevalent risk than obesity. In fact, our body's tendency to store fat when we overeat had survival value for our ancestors over millennia of episodic food scarcity.

This national preoccupation with weight is a mirror for our metaphysical state of being. We are so concerned about our physical attractiveness, and our sex appeal, that there is little emphasis or discussion of our inner character or our spiritual development.

Books and talk show hosts will often ascribe to a higher recognition of the values of charity, kindness, and compassion. But our true insecurities revolve around how good we look.

The "beauty" business is a multi-billion-dollar industry. Besides cosmetics, clothes, and personal trainers, there are the beloved plastic surgeons and dermatologists. The public in general may not be aware of the situation, but of all health care practitioners, only dermatologists and plastic surgeons routinely do not accept the payments of HMOs as full compensation. They know quite well that individuals will gladly pay their full fees in order to become more attractive. We seem to be of two minds: talking about the beauty of compassion and charity while deep down we are more concerned about our physical attractiveness.

Clearly, obesity does represent an enormous risk to one's health and in this regard it reflects upon not only the individual involved but the financial burden to our health care system.

Diabetes, heart disease, and stroke are undisputed complications of this condition. Apparently, there is new data to implicate obesity as a potent risk for cancer as well. Obese individuals suffer from sudden death as a consequence of cardiac arrhythmias and pulmonary embolism at a rate that far exceeds the general population.

Obviously, we cannot dismiss the power of physical beauty. I am as fascinated by the esthetics of a beautiful individual as anyone. One must be aware, however, at how culturally biased this notion can be. One can observe how powerfully the media can influence, both consciously and subconsciously, one's attitude regarding art or fashion. The same clearly applies to our attitudes about physical beauty. I am quite sure that contemporaries of the seventeenth-century Dutch artist Peter Paul Rubens, who delighted in painting full-figured women, would find contemporary female obsession with being extremely thin to be both unappealing and rather amusing.

Physical beauty need not be dismissed by the spiritually enlightened. Many spiritual traditions acknowledge any form of beauty as a gift from God. The following is a Hebrew prayer (in English) that can be said upon viewing an individual, a sunset, or any natural sight: "Blessed art Thou our Lord our God, King of the Universe who has such as this in his World." It is a prayer of gratitude for the gifts of beauty in general, not praise for the individual themselves.

Likewise, the enjoyment of sensual pleasures can be regarded as a spiritual gift. Kabbalistic writers have referred to men as "God's taste buds" in the world. This applies not only to the perception of beauty, but to the act of exercising our own taste buds—eating!

It is the failure to see past the outer veneer of face and form, it is the obsession with the physical at the expense of all else that is so damaging to our sense of being.

There may be a multitude number of reasons why someone becomes obese: genetics and metabolic processes certainly cannot be discounted. Other factors include the effects of advertising on creating a demand for products, the tendency to indulge one sensory modality (taste) when others have been deprived. The emotionally soothing effects when certain carbohydrate loads stimulate the release of serotonin and dopamine in our brains.

The simple cause of obesity is the ingestion of more calories than are utilized for metabolic processes. Logically speaking, reducing intake and/or increasing the burning of calories will accomplish the goal. The answer to this simple equation, however, is not so simple.

For many, it is slipping into habitual patterns of behavior. We are used to eating a certain amount and choosing those foods with higher caloric content. For many, it is simply eating when we are multitasking. We seem to attempt to do too much at one time. Eating becomes an event that takes place while we are doing other things—reading, writing, and speaking to others. Our lack of attention tends to drive us to eat more than we realize.

Religious traditions that emphasize prayer before meals can offer us a glimpse into a practical method of increasing awareness. It forces us to stop the automatic process of eating what appears to our eyes, nose, and mouth as tasty. It allows us to be mindful of the activity we are about to begin.

Hopefully, this mindfulness will continue throughout our meal. Being aware of each forkful . . . being present as we chew . . . being aware of the tastes of the food itself. All these activities will very likely allow us to experience our meals at a higher level, to actually taste what we are eating. Eating can become what it clearly should always have been—a sensual experience. Very likely, as well, we will eat more slowly, allowing our brain's signals for satiety (fullness) to be satisfied at lower quantities of food than previously.

The metaphysical and spiritual approach is also the healthy approach: Eat less, enjoy more, lose weight.

Perhaps our individual tendency to become obese is another test for us. It challenges us to take charge of our own lives, to act mindfully, to utilize our free will to make choices that will be in our best interest. The challenge to control our food choices carries over into the rest of our lives. We can accept our role not only in cocreating the universe, but in cocreating ourselves.

Part VII

Dr. Steve's Prescriptions for Calling Forth Your Inner Meta-Physician

Since the beginning of Creation—a piece of the world has been waiting for your soul to purify and repair it. And your soul, from the time it was first emanated and conceived, waited above to descend to this world and carry out that mission.

—Rabbi Menachem Schneerson

26

Twenty-seven Ways to Embrace Your Inner Meta-Physician

There are only two ways to live your life, one as if nothing is a miracle, the other as if everything is, I choose the latter.

—Albert Einstein

Many of us find our way to metaphysical wisdom and understanding after traumatic events that awaken our souls to search for life's deeper meanings. You can give yourself a head start by starting your own metaphysical journey now. You don't have to wait for a challenge or a catastrophe to bring out your higher self. Here are my prescriptions for tapping into your inner meta-physician.

ACKNOWLEDGE THE INNATE DESIRE TO MAKE SENSE OF REALITY

We all, on some level, want to know why life is the way it is and how to get a grip on all that is going on around us. This urge to understand may arise from a primal fear of disorder, death, and suffering. It could date back to ancestral memories of the time when we were threatened by who or what might be lurking behind the nearest tree or rock, or perhaps behind our back. Survival meant understanding the "rules of the game." Over the millennia, religion has partially filled this role, at least as it has served to alleviate the ultimate fear of death and dissolution. Science, as well, has arisen to uncover the mysteries of the physical universe. Never forget that your personal inquiry into the nature of your own existence is as valuable as any scientific theory and any religious doctrine. You are a child of the universe and you are endowed with the capacity and privilege of following your own path. If you put effort into an ongoing inquiry, you will reap the benefits of your endeavor. Seeking the reason for your life, and your purpose for being here, is a noble journey.

ACKNOWLEDGE THE VALUE OF SKEPTICISM VERSUS BLIND FAITH

I would be deeply gratified if this book serves you, but please feel no obligation to adopt the insights in this book or any other for that matter. In fact, do not believe everything you read or hear. Be an open-minded skeptic. Remember, every bit of data and information that assaults your senses has already been filtered through the lens of others—whether it's on TV, the Internet, magazines, film, or over coffee with a friend. Everyone has their own particular bias. Because both our conscious and subconscious minds are constantly engaged in the process of acting out programs from the past and present, it is possible to be affected by the pain, suffering and mythologies of others because these are derived from childhood or perhaps even past life influences. Just keep in mind that you must learn to self-filter; don't automatically believe everything you hear, even if it comes from a dear friend or loved one.

By the same token, it would be foolish to deny the possibility of extraordinary experiences when you hear of them through sources that are reliable and sincere. Listen with an open mind and heart to others. Your silence is often the window to wisdom. Be cautious as well. Some are motivated by profit, always selling something, or someone, as the guru or expert.

We live in a world that revels in questioning authority figures as well as grand and powerful institutions. That is often a reasonable and justified approach to exploring what is real. Large pharmaceutical companies are powerful corporate entities with billions of dollars to spend on research, development, promotion and advertising. They can help you heal but can also seduce your into believing your life depends on a certain medicine. Is the alternative approach the more honorable? Not necessarily. I've seen advertising that plays off the public's natural fears of disease, of being taken advantage of by large pharmaceutical companies, and of the deep desire to find safer and more natural approaches to health and healing. Having researched and explored some of these issues, I am amazed by the sheer skill of salesmanship in the false advertising I've discovered. The tactics often utilize infomercials and the Internet and often cleverly characterize traditional approaches as unhealthy, or even aligned with a conspiracy to trick and defraud the public. It is frighteningly persuasive.

So seek evidence for your beliefs. Certainly explore all sources of information including friends, professionals and the internet. Take a balanced approach and be sure to maintain an equally skeptical attitude toward so-called "natural" and "alternative" therapies as to the more traditional approaches. Seek the best information and be willing to follow the wisdom of your body's reaction to everything. You are unique and your responses to any therapy, traditional or alternative, may be as unique as you are.

RELIGION IS A CHOICE

If you were born into a religious family, this may seem rather radical, or perhaps even sacrilegious. If you are devout in your faith, you might even find it offensive. But the truth is that religion comes to us through a series of specific dogmas and doctrines from a historical/cultural and political perspective. You may regard your religion as the ultimate truth, and many in our Western culture look to Christianity as the absolute source of spiritual wisdom. Yet if you were born in

Tibet you would very likely regard Buddhism the same way. Or if you were from Calcutta, Hinduism would be your likely religious inheritance. Or if you were born in Damascus, Islam would seem true to you. So is "truth" more likely a function of where you were born and to which family? An example is the following: Idolatry is unacceptable in the Jewish faith because Jews are taught to experience God as an invisible force in the universe that guides them. God is evoked through prayer, song, chanting, and worship—but never via an image. Catholics, on the other hand, see Jesus as the son of God and speak to Christ through intermediaries such as Mary and a host of Saints who can be found as icons and holy art in Churches. Protestants on the other hand see Jesus as Lord and call upon him only, not paying much mind to Mary or the Saints of the Catholic tradition. While some branches of Christianity focus on him via the cross and holy images, others only permit the cross as a reminder of their relationship to Jesus. Hindus experience God in the same way, yet call to the Divine through worship of holy icons. Their Gods have multiples names, purposes, and incarnations. Pagans worship a Goddess as their main deity, and typically couple her with the Male Divine. Nature and natural cycles is a major focal point of worship. The point is, every faith has its own protocol and ways it calls to the Divine. This is a fact. But is any one faith ultimately true, while the others false? No! Thus, your religious path can be regarded as a "choice" rather than ultimate truth. If you find your truth in religion, go for it, but take care not to criticize or disrespect those who don't share your beliefs. Think of various religions as "languages." Perhaps there is one language that is clearer to you than another? Or perhaps you are interested in more than one? Somehow the concept of language carries less emotional power than that of religion. People are more likely to respect a different language than a different religion. Yet perhaps if they would regard religion as they do language, there would be far less hate in this world. Languages are optional. Each is regarded as capable of finding and describing truth. So, too, with different religions. While spirituality offers enlightenment, religion can sometimes be too mired in politics and protocol. While all religions teach a doctrine akin to the golden rule of doing unto others as one would have done to oneself, somehow it is only applied to individuals who share their own particular brand of dogma or belief. "Do unto others" does not truly apply to the "other" who is different in belief. When religion becomes the source of dividing people against each other, of fostering animosity and hatred, then it is time to acknowledge that a major fault line has been exposed. Under such circumstances it may be prudent to seek spiritual answers rather than those provided by institutionalized religion.

CONSIDER THE HEALING ASPECTS OF RELIGION

That said, there are soulful and spiritual aspects to religion that can truly feed the soul. On one level, it can serve as a tremendous source of comfort for individuals to gather together for spiritual enlightenment. Just the gathering, with the intention of sharing compassion, love, and connection with others, is tremendously healing. Prayer, for example, can lower stress and lower blood pressure. The value of ritual and community offered by religion can allay human suffering. It can help people know they truly are not alone. It can give a sense of an extended, like-minded family. Walking into a place where people know you—and you feel acknowledged and cared for—can truly be empowering. Religious services give us a place to go, to be ourselves, and to learn. Hopefully they help uplift and heal us. Religion provides rituals for life's rites of passage: from birth to entering a covenant by baptism, bris, or circumcision, confirmation, marriage, and death. Religious individuals do not have to create methods and protocols for each of life's transitions—they are already there for them to follow. By the same token, our world is filled with nonreligious ways to bring healing and spirituality in your life through group participation—this can include volunteering, community service, and simply being an active and helpful neighbor.

FAMILIARIZE YOURSELF WITH SOME OF THE LITERATURE REGARDING THE PARANORMAL

Just enter any of today's grand bookstores and make your way to the spirituality sections. New Age, "metaphysics," religion, philosophy—all are there to challenge you, to expand your consciousness. Allow time to take a break. Shut off the cell phones and e-mails. Forget the frenetic pace of our multitasking culture. Get lost. Browse science books that are written for the layman. The newest notions of biologic and physical reality are as counterintuitive and mind-blowing as any New Age creation. No one understands all the metaphysical ramifications of quantum and relativity theory. No one understands the origin of life. No one understands how our universe began, or why? Science is at the center of where metaphysical speculation begins. I frequently walk out with several books on science, others on life after death, reincarnation, quantum theory, Kabbalah, and Buddhist psychology or meditation. I find no contradictions or confusion here. Each bit of revealed truth contributes to the master mix of thought. Come with an open mind and a hunger for knowledge. Rise to the occasion by further educating yourself on metaphysical and healing topics, by continually challenging your mind to the possibility of the world that cannot be seen through the five senses alone. Can anyone prove that God or the soul exists, or that there is a higher purpose for existence? Should this dissuade or discourage further exploration? After all, it has been said that absence of proof is not the same as proof of absence. Just because there is no answer does not mean we should stop asking the questions. In fact, it only encourages us to do more. Mystery is present as much in science as it is in spirituality. Don't fear any of it. Explore the evidence for clairvoyance and psychic abilities, remote-viewing, reincarnation, near-death experience (NDE), after-death communication (ADC), and the medium experience before you try to reject it or shrug it off. You may be amazed at the world that opens to you and the new understanding it will bring.

READ THE BEST AND MOST REPUTABLE LITERATURE

Look for titles created by noteworthy authors. To begin with, seek literature by rational, highly educated individuals who offer their own experiences and evidence for the validity of otherwise dubious subjects. Many of these began their investigations from the position of deep skepticism and have applied a rational "scientific" approach to these subjects. At the same time, do not be afraid to buy books by authors who inspire or move you in some way. Use your intuition in selecting what strikes you as interesting. Also, reread what you have already read. There are numerous times when rereading material brings totally new insight. Also be careful not to only read what you have underlined. Too often I find a sentence of immense importance that I failed to underline, just next to one that I did. Strange how coming to a word or thought at a particular time will lead to such a unique experience and reaction.

GET OUT OF YOUR HEAD ...

Consider the *physical brain* and *conscious mind*. Are they one and the same? Do they exist in an interrelated physical universe or is the conscious mind like the Internet—connecting us to all other beings, the universe, and some cosmic God force the way a search engine seems to connect us to the world? Explore notions of the nature of mind and consciousness, and its relationship to the possibility that it can exist separate from the physical brain. If the concept that consciousness is a primary constituent of the universe itself is a possibility, then this would mean we are connected to all "that is." And this would allow us to see ourselves as a small element in the web of beings that exist as well. It would also mean that we don't have to seek an explanation for its origin. It just exists, as gravity does. And yet any mystery calls forth our desire to understand it. If consciousness is a part of the universe then why would we believe we alone possess it? And furthermore, if consciousness is a natural constituent of the universe then it would strongly suggest that there is an ultimate Consciousness—perhaps another name for God.

TAKE A SOULFUL APPROACH

What do we know of the soul? Is it a free creation of our imagination? Is it the product of wishful thinking, a powerful desire not to dissolve into the abyss of nonbeing? Perhaps it is worth considering that there is a spiritual component to living things. Can science study it, measure it, and analyze it? Of course not, yet there are those deeply personal yet powerfully compelling experiences that we have examined in this book. The near-death experience, after-death communication, apparitions, reincarnation tales, the medium experience all lend strong credence to the concept that an aspect of our selves survives and extends beyond the physical body. Buddhists deny the notion of a soul that reincarnates as an intact entity. Instead they recognize a consciousness that evolves and changes from life to life. Still, they recognize that karmic forces play a role in how our sacred contracts are expressed in any one lifetime.

But is the soul identical to the mind? An enlightened answer from a medium I know seems to address this question best. When asked to give his thoughts on the matter, medium Artie Hoffman went deep within to listen to his Higher Self, or perhaps his spiritual guide. His response was clearly not derived from his own mind. His response was this, "The soul manifests and observes, the mind creates and reacts." This most profound of statements is consistent with the belief that the soul enters the developing organism, merges with the physical brain to create the mind, but otherwise "sits out the dance." The merged mind is then in charge throughout the lifetime of the individual. It creates reality through its own perceptions, then reacts to its own creation. It strongly suggests that it is capable of creating alternative scenarios, of viewing its life in different ways and through a variety of lenses. The awareness that we have choice in the matter is crucial to our evolving. We can choose how we regard the events of our lives. We can choose whether we dwell in despair and negativity or seek to understand reality as ultimately offering us opportunities to grow and heal. This power to create our own reality is the gift of the soul to the evolving mind. It is very likely that many of our physical ailments result from conflicts between our mind, the soul that birthed it and aspects of our physical brain.

Dis-ease represents the lack of peaceful coexistence and integration of all aspects of our selves. Dis-ease, of course, leads inevitably to disease. Our souls are immortal, descending into the world of materiality in order to experience the challenges of our existence. It is for the purpose of growth and development, but it is risky business. The soul comes here without conscious memory of its true nature. Amnesia sets in when the mind forms from the conjunction of soul and brain. But there are hints of a grander nature to the soul. Some of us feel it, others intuit it, others listen for a small still voice.

SEE THE UNIVERSE AS EXPANSIVE

Consider the notion of a cosmic intelligence or universal mind, which finds its description in a variety of terms, including God. Our souls are a part of the essence of this universal force and they seek to reunite with that Source. This is what creates in us a hunger for religion and spirituality, a desire to know God. In this context, by knowing God, we know our true selves, as we are a part of this universal spirit. We can see ourselves as co-creators of this world. See ourselves as divine beings inhabiting physical "space suits." If we truly regarded ourselves as part of a higher cosmic mind, we would be incapable of causing others to suffer or to disparage ourselves, our minds, and our own bodies as anything but divinely inspired works of art.

BE AWARE THAT THERE WILL BE PEOPLE IN YOUR LIFE WHO DON'T "GET IT"

One of the greatest detractors of our true spiritual path can be, and might be, the people closest to us—if we let them. Some individuals in our lives may be highly critical and intolerant of our spiritual exploration. Complaints usually come from those who are deeply and blindly religious or committed atheists and closed-minded skeptics. And from those who are frightened by our newfound open-mindedness. Our spiritual awareness and flourishing consciousness may be a threat to the status quo and may be seen as something that shakes up the comfort zone of people close to us. If we are lucky, loved ones come around and accept—if not embrace—the journey we are on. Then again, there are those who never will and we must then accept the journey they are on. Remember, "To each his own!"

When we are first exposed to consciousness there is a tendency to become obsessed with the wisdom that flows from it. We are excited to tell *everyone* about what we have discovered. It is important to revel in self-expression and share your truth, but I suggest you do it in increments. And share yourself most fully when surrounded by like-minded souls who will celebrate your evolution. For example, if you vigorously proclaim your new insights regarding psychic or spiritual insights to your rather traditionally minded or observant religious parents, a scenario of conflict and contention may set in. They may not understand. Their negative reaction may set up a conflict between you, and within you, impairing the natural love that had previously flourished. A more subtle approach is to reveal—through your attitudes and behavior—a transformation of consciousness. This may actually stimulate them to inquire about your new state of being. By observing how your explorations have made you a spiritually more content and compassionate human being, all of those who know you may be curiously open to learning about your own path. The proof of any metaphysical concept should be in how it affects us in this lifetime. We can all be living examples of what an evolving consciousness can become.

EXPLORE THE FINDINGS OF CONTEMPORARY SCIENCE

Explore the wonder of this universe through exploring the latest findings in science. Science and spirituality are not in conflict. Despite what many people think—and despite the strange and bizarre beliefs of certain fundamentalist religious fanatics—science is not the enemy of spirituality. Many of our greatest scientists find inspiration for their life's work in the belief that there is a higher intelligence that underlies the nature of reality. This does not contradict the theory of evolution either. As a matter of fact, evolution is a completely spiritual concept. After all, aren't our souls evolving toward perfection? Why should the physical, biological world be any different? Biology, physics, cosmology are leading many scholars and scientists to view the universe as living, evolving, interactive,

and organic rather than inert and machine-like. Science is a primary tool of
metaphysical inquiry. Seek out the latest stories and studies on these topics. You
can easily find them on the Internet and reputable journals. You can even sign
up for "Google Alerts" on the topics that interest you most. It can become a truly
empowering experience to start paying attention to scientific topics in the news
and to expand your knowledge base.

EXAMINE YOUR OWN UNUSUAL EXPERIENCES

Have you ever thought you felt a deceased relative "around you"? Ever think
of someone and—they call you on the phone? Has someone you knew a long
time ago come into your mind and suddenly you run into that person or someone
who also knows that person? The "coincidences" of the universe are often our
spiritual path of synchronicity unfolding before our very eyes. Don't be afraid to
explore those experiences that have paranormal or spiritual elements. Be aware
that many of us harbor a fear of the unknown—particularly when it has to do
with these topics. I was somewhat surprised by how common this sentiment is,
even among otherwise sophisticated and well-educated individuals. Perhaps this
should be referred to as "meta-phobia"—the fear of exploring the nature of reality.

I suppose it is always difficult to relate to a phobia that we don't share. For
instance, my usual fear of heights might seem equally incomprehensible to someone who doesn't have it. Phobias in general are actually exaggerated fears of
something that has a core of truth to the fear. Fear of heights, for instance, makes
evolutionary sense on a moderate level. It clearly protected our ancestors from
calmly walking off cliffs. Perhaps fear of the metaphysical unknown represents a
similar warning—tread carefully when dealing with spiritual realms. There are
those who profess to understand the "dark side" of spirituality. It is also true that
nearly all mediums "protect" themselves before they enter a clairvoyant state
of consciousness. The so-called dark forces may literally be souls and spiritual
entities that remain confused and unenlightened about their true nature (i.e., a
ghost is typically seen as someone who is dead but does not realize it). The caveat
about playing with Ouija boards has to do with the lower-level energies that may
be earthbound, unable or unwilling to leave the addictions of the physical world,
despite their lack of a physical body. So perhaps some prudence is indicated when
exploring the world of spirit. But this warning does not have relevance to the
exploration for metaphysical truth. Truth should never be feared. On the contrary, living in an illusion makes little sense. How can we ever hope to acquire a
sense of peace and joy if we fear what is real? What seems odd and a little scary
at first can be the very same thing that expands your intuition and your ability
to merge the spiritual with the mundane in daily life. For example, imagine if
your loved ones on the "other side" truly were sending you messages as a way of
trying to help you. They may give hints about an illness you need to address, or
a job or relationship you need to pursue. One student was feeling very ill, with
lower-abdominal cramping. It was one year to the day of her father's death, so

she asked a meditation teacher to help her connect to his soul in a meditation. He came to her so strongly she could hear his actual voice and he *urged* her to go to the doctor and "listen to what the doctors tell you to do." She was resistant, but followed her father's advice. The final diagnosis was diverticulitis, which may have likely progressed to the point of possible perforation and peritonitis. The early treatment allowed her to avoid unnecessary complications. The messages may not always be as profound, and they may be mundane, but if we pay attention, we may be guided to better heath, well-being, and peace. For support and reinforcement, share these topics with trusted friends and associates. And seek out spiritual communities that "get" what your experience is all about. You can find similar examples in the writings of others and there are small groups and clubs around the world who gather like-minded people to discuss psychic phenomenon and metaphysical experiences.

ENCOURAGE OTHERS TO SHARE THEIR OWN PRIVATE EXPERIENCES

Just as you need a safe and sacred space in which to share your inner thoughts and feelings, it is a blessing to also provide that for others. Once you begin to open up to these kinds of experiences in your life, others will flock to you with their stories. That has been my unequivocal experience. Give them a safe, nonjudgmental opportunity to share. They may have suppressed some of them, out of fear of the negative reaction of others. Open the door to them, and it will open a door to healing for you as well. The purity of the exchange of such insights, experiences, and information between people who are sharing from their personal truth and reality is extremely powerful. It reflects the highest form of compassion and shared healing.

PUT THE CREDIBILITY QUOTIENT TO THE TEST

Obviously, you want to keep your open-minded skeptic on high alert as you open more to the depths of this spiritual experience. Be cautious not to seek out people who are "selling something" as your primary source of information at first. Over time you will learn to become more discerning, and you will learn to open and trust your intuition more. You will be able to discern the authentic experiences of those who have no incentive to fabricate anything. When this is still new to you, make sure you seek people who have had their own authentic spiritual and paranormal stories and are willing not just to share but who are open to the truth of their experiences. This is about personal exploration, and exchanges with those who could not possibly benefit by fabricating any such experience. For example, there is a club called "The Psychic Club" in Queens, New York. It was founded by a couple that lost an adult child and were seeking a way to connect with his soul. On the journey, they found a new awakening within themselves, something they could have never expected. They started calling like-minded people together to share similar personal experiences. Soon, people were connecting on a deep level. The cross-sharing of real-life experiences with psychic phenomena became a way of life for the founders and the many that would flock to the club each month. It was a sigh of relief, a feeling of having come home. Participants could stand before the group and announce, "My grandmother came to me in a dream last night," or "I am feeling my ex-husband around my house," and people in the audience would nod their heads in understanding.

FIND THE METAPHYSICAL BALANCE

While the credibility quotient is an excellent tool when dealing one on one directly with someone who has had a stirring spiritual experience, it may limit your understanding of paranormal/spiritual phenomenon to some extent—if it is related to someone other than the person you are discussing it with. Truth is, the farther away you are from such an unusual experience, the less likely you are to believe it to be true, or the less likely you are to have an immediate response that lets you know it is true. For example, if you are chatting with a friend at work and she relays a tale from someone else's life, it may be intriguing but may not be as powerful as if the person had shared it directly. This does not mean it did not really happen. It just means that when you are once or twice (or more) removed from the person who had the experience, the sharing of the incident may not stir you in the same way.

If your friend shares an experience about her husband, who had a dream that his mother was standing over his bed and awoke to a phone call letting him know she passed, it may give you the chills because your friend was in the same bed with him when he had the "dream" and received the call. But if she shares the same story about her husband's boss or something she saw on television, it may not have the same impact. However, if she said, "I was lying in bed with my husband last night when the phone rang. His mom had passed. He took the call and quietly shook his head. Then he told me he had just had a dream that she was standing over his bed. She must have come to say goodbye." Somehow, the latter brings the story home.

UNDERSTAND DEATH AS A TRANSITION

One of our greatest fears is that we, or someone we love, will die. We spend our days and nights trying to protect ourselves from the very threat that lurks around every corner. We lock our doors and windows, look over our children as they sleep, go to doctors when we feel a twinge of something uncomfortable. Many obsess over diet and exercise. Many consume enormous quantities of vitamins and supplements in the vain hope of escaping the ultimate fate of us all. Of course this does not imply that one should abandon good judgment about any of these topics. But perhaps a more moderate approach will provide the same long-term benefits without the unnecessary self-denial. Many of us feel we are staring death in the face at every turn—when we drive, fly in planes, sail in boats, go camping, swim the ocean. The list goes on. Our fear of death and our constant vigil to keep it at bay from our doorstep and our lives makes us neurotic and fearful. For all the time we spend guarding against it in daily living, we are not living at all. We are waiting for death and fearing its arrival. It drains the life force from us. Then, when death comes to someone we know, we deem it a tragedy. Indeed, loss of a loved one is a horrible experience for many of us. So, often we find ourselves wracked with pain and feel that sometimes life itself seems meaningless. If all of us, if everyone we know and care for, will die, what's the purpose of living in the first place? Ironically, the answer arises from the same statement. Because life is temporary, we need to enjoy every possible moment. When we have made our peace with death, we will not fear to engage life fully. When we accept that everyone we know and love will die, we will not hold back our expression of love and commitment in the here and now. If you can fully comprehend this, you will have achieved a great deal of the message of this book and will have made great strides in your personal metaphysical growth. You can *choose* how you regard death: as ultimate tragedy, or ultimate motivation to embrace life fully. Couple that with the powerful evidence for survival of the soul, and even the fear of never being with loved ones again is alleviated. We need to view death as a transition to another realm of consciousness. See it as the shedding of our human skin and you will gradually lose fear of it. Include in this understanding the death of situations, relationships, or jobs. It all means transition, metamorphosis and opportunity for growth.

CONSIDER THE CONCEPT OF KARMA AND REINCARNATION

If you were Hindu or Buddhist, Wiccan or raised with mystical Judaism, you would hold this world view as a natural part of the cycles of life. Certain faiths organically accept these concepts as part of their everyday being and they base their experience in the world on the understanding that they come into a lifetime with certain karmic debt to "burn off." Karma and reincarnation are twin concepts. The purpose of rebirth is to face karmic issues from past lives and to do a better job of doing the right thing, making choices that favor love over hate, compassion over abandonment, and goodness over evil. If we understand that our essence is that of an immortal soul, we can understand that each individual lifetime here is merely "survival weekend." Because we have the perspective of our one life only, we fail to comprehend how short any human lifetime truly is. From the perspective of eternity, whether we live nine weeks or ninety years makes little difference. Did we fulfill our mission here? That is a more significant question that we should all ask ourselves. As difficult as it may be to accept, perhaps a newborn child came into this world to live a short time in order for its parents to learn acceptance, compassion, and seek the healing touch of loved ones. Perhaps those young children with shortened lives were themselves advanced souls who sacrificed a lifetime through compassion for the needs of other souls.

If we can only come to the understanding that life is not supposed to be easy—that we take difficult courses in school to challenge us to learn more, that our lives here are just like that—then we are less likely to feel that we are the victims of outside forces. If we understand that we may have set ourselves up for difficulties before we incarnated here, then we have no one to "blame" at all. We can take responsibility for our lives. We can also come to accept that life is imperfect, for everyone. Perhaps we can come to terms with "managing imperfection" as our ultimate role here. We can also understand how the concept of healing has much greater implications than that of our physical bodies. Since we will all die, how can we speak about ultimate healing? The truth is that when we understand that healing means coming to terms with our fears, of seeking and striving to be our highest selves, then healing can occur even as our bodies are approaching death.

SEE THE LESSONS IN LIFE

Welcome to the big classroom known as life. Or, on rough days, "survival training." If we choose to see a higher purpose for the disappointments, devastations and heartache of our human lives it helps us make sense of some of the sadness and insanity that befalls us here on earth. If we know we are here to learn, then we can respect the lessons that are offered us—regardless of the pain. Feeling that pain and suffering are natural and unavoidable may not take the pain away. But it should give us a larger perspective by which to experience them—as triumphs when we learn our lessons well and can then move on. When we resist that which we are here to learn, we will continue to struggle and suffer from fear and confusion. If we regard life's difficulties as challenges our soul undertook for the purpose of spiritual growth and evolution, we have a better chance of getting through them without the additional suffering brought about by self-pity or the victim mentality. Understand the difference between pain and suffering. Pain is a natural part of human existence; the degree of suffering, however, becomes a personal choice. It all depends on how you regard the universe and your place in it. Acceptance of what is the fate of all humanity allows us to move through the quagmire of the dark emotions without getting stuck there. People who seek to avoid life's painful lessons often become addicts (whether addicted to alcohol and drugs or shopping) or they remain in a state of chronic dis-ease, which inevitably leads to physical ailments and failure to heal.

UNDERSTAND THAT EVOLUTION IS THE NATURE OF THE UNIVERSE

We are not meant to stand still or remain stagnant. In fact we have no choice about it—we are dying by the second. So if we come to terms with the flow of existence, we might just as well "jump in" rather than wait by the sidelines. We humans are meant to flow through life as if traveling on a journey, and the journey leads us from experience to experience. Our goal is not just to reach a destination, but to learn from and enjoy the process, that is the journey. Marriage is a great example of this. Married is not a static state of being. It is truly an evolving process, one which has a living organic quality to it. If it is continuously nurtured with love and consideration, it will flourish. It not, regardless of its auspicious beginning, it will undoubtedly fade and dissipate. Just as the most magnificent plant will surely fade and die without attention and care, the same is true of any relationship between individuals. This means that two people in love evolve together, individually as well as a partnership, and that their marriage becomes a living entity with its own inertia and energy. And just as our individual lives experience periods of positive and negative feelings such as joy and despair, the living nature of a marriage ensures that it will not be free of difficulties. And just as we attempt to understand and correct our individual challenges and sufferings, we pour our concerted energy into overcoming the challenges and obstacles which face our relationships. Sometimes these are successful and healing occurs. At other times, despite our best efforts, the relationships itself evolves into a different state of being. Separation is not necessarily the same as failure. Divorce is not the same as disease. Just as moving on in a career need not be regarded as a failure. Perhaps a relationship fulfilled its mission for a limited amount of time within the lives of its participants. Lessons were hopefully learned that will allow each to move on with greater healing and understanding of their unique paths.

Yet as with any living being, lack of sustenance will inevitably lead to its death. Failure to feed and nurture any relationship will doom its continuation. It has been said that marriage is meant to be a falling in love with one another, over and over. Yet love evolves as well. The rush of dopamine our brains experience with the early stages of romantic and sexual love inevitably fades. But if a deeper commitment and concern for the other person grows, marriage can continue to grow.

One's career aspirations and goals have the quality of a living, evolving process as well. Perhaps you set goals for your career when you were young. Then circumstances beyond your control derailed or sidetracked them. Perhaps you hit a "career wall" of some kind, or clashed with a particular boss. Perhaps you got fired and found yourself drifting in a sea of uncertainty. These were frightening and uncomfortable times. But they need to be viewed and interpreted as opportunities to transform and re-create yourself. Choose to view all dramatic changes as unexplored opportunities for growth and change. Perhaps it was your fault that you were fired. Perhaps it was a wake-up call that you needed to redirect yourself or refocus your energies. In any case, it does not have to be viewed as an ultimate tragedy. The mind, the spirit, and the body all require tune-ups, reevaluations, and attention. The care and feeding of the soul is of primary importance. We all need the love and attention of others but we do not have to sit back and wait—we can be there for ourselves first and foremost.

UNDERSTAND THAT LIFE'S TRAGEDIES ARE NOT PUNISHMENT FOR SIN

Nothing is worse for your health—mental, physical and spiritual—then the belief that your burdens, troubles, and sad situations in life are punishment for "sins" you have committed. Despite what some powerful religious doctrines proclaim, I do not accept the notion that I am inherently a sinner. Am I capable of committing a sinful act? Of course. I have free will like any other human being. But the ability to commit a sin does not make me inherently a "sinner." I would rather choose to believe the Kabbalistic concept that I and all of creation contain a spark of divinity within us. Certainly the physical shell that surrounds that spark adds an enormous challenge to the notion of choosing to be God-like. But once again, I can choose to not see myself as inherently a sinner, merely a human being with the capacity to choose good or evil. The belief that someone is inherently a sinner is a concept that has the capacity to truly make people sick—physically, mentally, and spiritually. To believe that something bad has happened because of a sin you unknowingly committed or naively perpetuated can cast a pall on your life in more ways than one. As a physician, I believe that this kind of belief system is damaging for mind, body, and spirit. It perpetrates the myth that an individual deserves to suffer, be unhappy, unsuccessful. It establishes a vicious cycle of self-defeat, lack of self-esteem followed by lack of effort, which confirms their low expectations for themselves. It weakens the immune system. There are numerous examples in which a community has imposed its judgment upon the inherent value and goodness of one of its members. The affected individual, accepting the verdict, will often comply and literally crawl up into a ball and die. There may or may not be any active disease process that can be identified. Yet the power of self-belief cannot be denied. In reality, tragedy and difficulty are not by-products of your sins. They are extraordinary opportunities for overcoming and learning. To soften the tough times, seek the gifts of joy and beauty that replenish the soul. Realize that God manifests grace through the kindness, love, and compassion of other people.

CONSIDER WE LIVE IN A BROKEN WORLD

If we understand, from the start, that it is the world that is broken and needs repair we have a greater chance to rise to the occasion to help heal ourselves and our world. Trying to find wholeness in an incomplete world is a daunting task if we believe that we are the only ones with problems and the only one whose lives are in disrepair. We tend to look at the lives of others and imagine that the grass is greener and their lives are easier. But everyone had their cross to bear and their burdens to lift. The universe itself is simply not complete. If it were, if would not seem so broken and in need of human attention and help. I believe strongly this is one of the most important reasons for our being. We cannot *start out* feeling whole because we live in a world that is a work in progress. Makes sense that our incomplete universe would bring forth individuals who feel that sense of incompleteness in everyday life. It is that sense of something missing that moves us to fill in the blanks, right the wrongs, and correct the imbalances. When Kabbalists are asked where is God in times of tragedy and suffering, their answer is simple: "God sends other people to do His work." Taking on the challenge of living in this world with full consciousness, and helping the world right itself as we get our own lives in order, is a mission for those of us who are blessed enough to understand the truth of our existence. This is the definition of true healing. See yourself as a co-creator with Divinity.

LET IN GOD IN HUMAN FORM

We tend to look at the Divine being as masculine or feminine in nature. Or in other traditions, see the ultimate nature of Divinity as formless or beyond description. But God comes to us in many forms, including human representatives who carry the divine spark within. There are humans all around us who are emissaries of God and the light of the divine. There may be divine beings here on earth whose mission is to assist humanity in its struggles. Of course we could criticize them for not doing enough, as there are plenty of examples where help is needed. Yet they are not here to take over for us. We are the primary movers on the physical plane and must take credit or blame for the way the world is. It is interesting that Hindu, Buddhist, and Kabbalistic traditions elevated souls who have graduated from the cycle of reincarnation but who chose to assume human form in order to assist in the functioning of this world. For example, Kuan Yin is a popular Bodhisattva in the Chinese Buddhist tradition who is regarded historically as a kind princess who once walked the earth and died cruelly. Given the opportunity to reach nirvana, she decided instead to stay on earth until the last tear of human suffering has dried. The Christian concept of Christ dying for the sins of humanity reflects a similar notion of self-sacrifice in order to teach lessons of growth and healing. Be open to the possibility that divine beings are all around us. The stranger in the store or the beggar on the street may be examples. They may not have wings but they have spirit—and plenty of it. They will share it with you without condition if you allow it. They will come to you in times of trouble and confusion. They will be there to catch you when you fall. Understand that in the midst of suffering, others offer their love as Divine representatives.

UNDERSTAND HEALING AS A METAPHOR FOR
THE HUMAN EXPERIENCE

If everything were perfect, we would have no work to do here on earth. We would ramble about the Garden, enjoying nature's bounty, never stepping out to take the risk of tasting what is unknown or take the challenge of learning about ourselves and the world around us. If things were good all the time we would be stagnant, unmoving, stuck in a place where there is no life force to keep us evolving as we must, in order to learn all the lessons of our human experience. I have said it before and it's worth repeating: Healing can be seen as a description of both the process and goal of all life. Healing becomes a perfecting of our souls, developing our minds as well as maintaining our physical bodies. If we view ultimate perfection as being whole or healed, then humanity will always fall short of that lofty state of being. But any activity that gets us closer to wholeness is healing. If we define *ignorance* as a lack of knowledge of any kind, then learning becomes healing. If we tend to be selfish and less than loving toward others then acquiring compassion and empathy is a form of healing. Because our souls have incarnated here, we remain incomplete. Any effort to achieve growth becomes healing, and the purpose of our incarnation. Healing means viewing ourselves as part of the universe. It transcends the traditional notion of the physical body and must incorporate the mind and soul as well. Do not despair when you feel uneasy in mind, body, or spirit. See it as an opportunity to heal!

BE OPEN TO EXPLORING ALTERNATIVE OR COMPLEMENTARY APPROACHES TO HEALING

There is no need, ever, to live in an either/or state of mind. Our universe is ripe with options and opportunities for healing so no one should ever feel that traditional medicine is the only option—nor should we swing to the other extreme and refuse all allopathic care and use only alternative or a "holistic" health approach in its place. Extreme positions of any kind usually lead to problems because life is a fluid, constantly changing state of being. We must be willing to try new approaches, but be equally vigilant to potential benefits or adverse reactions. At its best, healing is much more of an art than a science. Surely, scientific knowledge is crucial to understanding the functioning of the physical being. Yet it is an art in the sense that it is constantly changing and evolving, even within one individual. The best practitioners are the most humble. These are individuals who understand the enormous complexity of every living being and feel deeply gratified and relieved when patients improve. Yes, relieved when anyone gets better! The greatest healing and the best healers understand that what is required is a balance. It is important to check out what is available, while maintaining an appropriate skeptic's view when it comes to unsubstantiated or unstudied claims. While you never want to jump blindly into an unknown and unproven treatment, proper research and consumer holistic health education can help you make wise decisions about complementary treatments. For example, if you are dealing with a serious health issue, you want to test and monitor it with your allopathic doctor, and then seek therapies that complement or aid your existing treatment, or ease its adverse effects. For example, many cancer patients lessen the effects of chemotherapy by enjoying a Reiki session while resting at home or in the hospital. A Reiki practitioner offers a style of hands-on healing that is like a prayer filled with healing energy. One woman I know had a pain just off center of the middle of her chest. One doctor said it was asthma-related costochondritis from severe coughing. An osteopath said she had two ribs sticking together. Her primary doctor said she had to follow cardiac testing protocol, allergy testing, and GI testing just to "rule anything out." She did all that, but also called in a trained shamanic practitioner, who took her on a "metaphysical journey" to visit the roots of her pain in what the shamans call "the lower world." In discovering there were "stuffed" emotions in that area she was able to begin releasing them by understanding their source. A *shaman* is the traditional medicine man or woman in the Incan tradition. Calling in a spiritual practitioner, enhanced the help she was getting from other physicians, helped her deal with—and heal—the ways her imbalance of mind/body and spirit had manifested itself over time in her physical form.

HONOR MEDICINE FOR ALL ITS CONTRIBUTIONS TO OUR HEALTH

God works through penicillin, too. Some people these days reject the notion of the healing power of traditional medicine. They focus on the politics and costs of treatments, on HMOs and insurance issues. But medicine today has changed our lives immeasurably. Just imagine, thirty years ago, most cancer was considered incurable. People would get a diagnosis, a doctor would tell them how long they have and they would go home and die on schedule. Of my patients today, many are in their 70s, 80s, and 90s, and have implanted pacemakers and defibrillators, many have had coronary bypass surgery and/or stents, others have been treated for breast, colon, or prostate cancer. All of them would be dead today without traditional, allopathic medical care.

Visit an old cemetery and take note of the age of death of many of the inhabitants. You may be shocked to observe how many were young children or women in the childbearing years. Such occurrences are fortunately rather rare today—for a good reason. Today's advances keep millions of cancer patients alive for long periods of time with good quality of life. AIDS and its treatment is a prime example. Once a death sentence, many people continue to have a good life after diagnosis because of the special treatment available in this country. Illness has taught us to care more about our immune systems and refine our lifestyles. Advances in medicine and surgery have helped millions upon millions of people deal with an illness, rather than succumb to it. Do not reject the tremendous achievements of science and technology in the relief of physical suffering. Rather, integrate them within a broader context, which includes a holistic perspective.

CONSIDER PRAYER AND MEDITATION

It is said that prayer is about talking to the Divine and meditation is about contemplating the answers. You don't have to be a mystic or a monk to pray and/or meditate every day. Many, many studies have shown that prayer helps people heal, this includes distant healing as well as personal meditation on one's own immune system. But you do not need a study to know this. Not religious?

You do not have to address your prayers to God to have a response. Many people consider themselves spiritual but not religious, and yet call upon the ancient tools of religious worship to help in everyday life in a nondenominational way. Explore meditation and prayer as vehicles for opening your intuitive nature and training your mind. We inhabit a culture that is obsessed with training the body but ignores the mind. Make mind and spirit training a priority and you will open up the gates to many treasures—including well-being, peace of mind, a sense of control over your life, and, yes, even a little bliss here and there.

EMBRACE THE ROLE OF META-PHYSICIAN

It is a gift of human awareness. The meta-physician in all of us clamors to be free. We need to honor our need to know. Self-awareness, our knowledge of who we are and why we are here, is crucial to the task at hand—to heal ourselves as we heal the world.

Enjoy the process of uncovering the nature of reality!

27

Labyrinth or Maze: Which Path Will You Choose?

Life can only be understood backwards, but it must be lived forwards.
—Søren Kierkegaard

We are all destined to follow a path that is uniquely our own. This does not mean the path will be straight or smooth. It does not mean that it will be effortless or easy. In fact, paradoxically, our lives only begin to make sense when we *expect* to encounter bumps, potholes, detours, and obstacles.

Does that last statement seem unusually depressing and pessimistic? Not if we understand that the purpose of our lives here is to provide our souls, our Higher Selves, with an opportunity to learn and grow, to uncover and proceed along our own path. Because as French Jesuit priest and paleontologist Teilhard de Chardin noted, "We are not human beings having a spiritual experience, but rather spiritual beings having a human experience."

Each individual path will be ours, as unique as our own DNA, and as personal as our view on life. But there is no satellite computer navigation system that will tell us where to turn, how to go. We must assume that role ourselves. We must exercise our free will and trust our inner voice as well. And we must rise to the effort with courage and enthusiasm.

Accepting that responsibility and choosing our unique path will be a source of our own empowerment. It is important to make a fundamental choice about the *kind* of path we will take and *how* to take it. This means choosing to see our lives as a maze or a labyrinth. The distinction between the two is significant. A maze can appear confusing and dangerous, with many blind passages and dead-end cul-de-sacs. A maze can lead us into an abyss of confusion and despair. It can frustrate, fragment us, bring us to the brink of dis-ease and disease. In contrast, a labyrinth may *seem to be a maze* at first but is not. It may appear at times to stymie us in our pursuit of a peaceful and loving life. But these are only temporary, minor obstacles, placed before us to teach us to evolve and heal. Ultimately, upon looking back, we come to understand that each bump in the road, each blind curve was absolutely essential for our journey.

Each one of our lives may appear to be a maze. It is quite easy to become confused, frustrated, even depressed about it. Yet through our intention, attitude, and approach to the journey, we can turn around when we realize that the blind alley we've stumbled into was a temporary detour along our own personal labyrinth.

Our state of mind and our attitude reflects greatly upon *how* we experience our journey. Will we face each obstacle with a calm understanding of the purpose of life? Will we accept them as painful but necessary opportunities for growth? Or will we be swallowed up by self-pity, despair, and worry? Will we seek to find and express gratitude for life's gifts or will we see ourselves as unfortunate victims of life's lottery?

My practice of medicine has provided me with many examples of the power of the choices we make and the paths we choose. I have treated numerous patients who wore their life's stresses like an anchor around their neck. They rarely smiled. They sat slumped over in my examination room. Their voices were somber and monotone. Their complaints were often the physical manifestations of their emotional state of being. When I would question them about their lives I uncovered that they had many potential sources of pleasure—friends, children, grandchildren, religious affiliations, organizations, and clubs. They seemed, however, to be reluctant to admit that they had reasons to be grateful for their lives. They downplayed their pleasures, focused on their suffering. They regarded themselves as victims of life's unfairness, and their physical complaints paralleled these feelings.

When I could get them to acknowledge the episodes of joy and fulfillment in their lives, many would smile and visibly change their posture and voice. They would instantly seem lighter and, not surprisingly, their symptoms miraculously improved as well. "Take 'that' prescription home with you," I would joke.

After observing themselves, and their attitudes, many patients would come to understand how their state of mind was contributing to their physical ailments. Others, however, would return with the same complaints, over and over. Habits of any kinds—even poor choices—are not easily changed. But they can be. It takes awareness and courage, however, to do so. This is essential to any process of healing.

Viktor Frankl, in his classic study of Holocaust survivors in *Man's Search for Meaning*, wrote about the capacity and ability of some concentration camp inmates to grasp at the tiniest signs of life around them: a sunrise through the slits of their decrepit cabins, the first sounds of birds in the spring, a glimmer of a new bud on a tree limb. These were spiritual sustenance for them. They were determined to survive in spite of the attempts to destroy them psychologically as well as physically. They created mind games for themselves, visualizing their lives before and, hopefully, after the camps.

Rabbi Joseph Gelberman, a Kabbalistic Master and founder of the New Synagogue in New York, lost his wife and young child in the Holocaust, yet has based his life on the premise that we are meant to be joyous, excited about life, and loving—despite what hardships may come. He often quotes from Psalm 23, "Yea, though I walk through the valley of the shadow of death, I will fear no evil," and talks about how continuing the journey despite life's difficulties is the point. Giving up is not an option.

Rabbi Harold Kushner commented on the next phrase of Psalm 23, which states, "for Thou art with me." He noted that God does not promise that life is fair or easy. Only that we would not have to face it alone.

We who have so much to be grateful for also seem to fixate on the darkness. To *see* the light is a choice. To call it into your life takes an act of will, sometimes in the face of overwhelming pain. But it is a choice we can live with.

Glossary

After-death Communication (ADC): A term first used by Bill Guggenheim and Judy Guggenheim in *Hello From Heaven!* (New York: Bantam Books, 1995).

The anthropic principle: A concept that the existence of the physical universe as we know it is incredibly unlikely based on the laws of probability and the magnitude of multiple physical constants.

Baal Shem Tov: Born Israel ben Eliezer in 1696 and died in 1760, he was a force for embracing the mystical, emotional aspects of Kabbalsitic thought and establishing a living form of religious practice. The name means "Master of the Good Name" or the four letter name of God in Hebrew, which is never pronounced.

Bimah: Platform from in a Jewish synagogue from which the Torah is read.

CAM: Complementary and alternative medicine.

Cognitive dissonance: A mental discomfort arising from conflicting beliefs of attitudes held simultaneously. Described by Leon Festinger in 1957.

Dark night of the soul: A spiritual crisis referenced to Spanish mystic and priest St. John of the Cross.

Evolutionary biology and psychology: Accepted concept of the origin and development of all life. It evaluates particular traits, both physical and psychological, as providing some benefit to the species over time. What may appear to be a "negative" trait may only reflect an excessive degree of what is most likely beneficial to the survival of the species. An example would be the tendency to "worry" about everything. In moderation it produces survival, in excess, neurosis.

"God Is Dead": From the cover story "Is God Dead?" *Time Magazine*, April 8, 1966. Describes the attitude of several contemporary theologians and the cultural ramifications that ensued.

Holy Sparks: Refers to a Kabbalistic concept first introduced by Rabbi Isaac Luria in the sixteenth century and reiterated by the founder of Hasidism, Baal Shem Tov, in the eighteenth century. Refers to the notion that after Creation, the incipient world shattered, leaving sparks of Divinity enclosed in all physical forms. Through good works and through the following of commandments humankind, can contribute to the repair (*tikkun*) and rededication of the physical world through the raising of Holy Sparks. This is seen as a gift from God since mankind is allowed to participate in this process of cocreation.

Kabbalah Centre: An incorporated worldwide educational nonprofit organization operated by the Berg family with controversial interpretation and formulation of Kabbalistic precepts into their own branded version.

Kalama Sutra: Tells the story of Buddha's visit to the village of Kesaputta, where he was greeted by the inhabitants, known as the Kalamas. The Kalamas ask the Buddha whose teachings they should follow. In response, he delivered a sutta that serves as an entry point to Buddhist beliefs to those unconvinced by revelatory experiences. His response, quoted in the opening of this book, has become the Buddhist charter on free thought.

Kavanah: This refers to the intention or inner feeling that accompanies prayer or good deeds known as mitzvoth (plural of mitzvah).

Leap of faith: From Danish philosopher and writer Soren Kierkegaard, to describe the Christian experience, not based exclusively upon rational inquiry.

Mitzvot: According to Jewish law there are specifically 613 mitzvot (commandments) that God gave to the people of Israel. These include the "Ten Commandments."

Monkey mind or monkey chatter: A concept referred to in many meditations and books. While it is attributed to Buddhist origins, and part of the modern Buddhism vernacular, the source is unclear. It refers to the constant jumping from thought to thought without pause or rational connection, similar to a monkey in a zoo leaping around its cage. It is the goal of meditation to "tame" this pattern of the mind.

Near-death experience (NDE): A term first coined by Raymond Moody Jr. in *Life After Life: The Investigation of a Phenomenon—Survival of Bodily Death* (New York: Bantam Books, 1975).

Nocebo: It is the opposite of the placebo effect. It represents an undesirable response or reaction to an "inert" or inactive pill. It, too, demonstrates the power of the mind to affect the body.

Psychoneuroimmunolgy: The relationship between mind and body by evidence of scientific testing and the discovery of circulating peptides that connect the mind, brain, and the immune system. Referenced to Robert Ader and Nicholas Cohen of the University of Rochester who coined the term in 1975 (Wikipedia reference). Also used by Candace Pert, *Molecules of Emotion* (New York: Scribner, 1997).

Senescence: The natural process resulting in the loss of individual cells' ability to divide and therefore renew the organism itself. The result is an increased risk for disease and ultimately death.

Shattering of vessels: Elaborated by Kabbalistic mystic, Rabbi Isaac Luria (1554–1572), it speaks to the notion of an incomplete creation, the falling of divine sparks into the physical universe, which became hidden in shells (*kelipot*). Humankind can be a cocreator with God by liberating the holy sparks of divinity that exist in these shells through the performance of good deeds (mitzvoth).

Spiritual dimension to reality (SDR): A concept in which a variety of personal experiences—including a near-death experience, after-death communication, apparitional experience, psychic or medium experience—brings to an individual a deep knowing that a spiritual dimension to reality truly exists. This knowledge then forms the basis for their metaphysical belief system.

Talis: A fringed prayer shawl, worn by observant Jews during morning services, Torah services, and on Yom Kippur.

The Ten Plagues: Part of the traditional Passover Seder, these represent the incremental punishing of the Pharaoh and the Egyptians in their refusal to release the Israelite slaves. A drop of wine is removed from the glass of the participants in the Seder for each plague enumerated in order to show compassion for the suffering of those same Egyptians who held the Israelites in bondage. *The Haggadah*—the Passover guidebook—clearly states that one is not to rejoice in the suffering of others. It is a symbolic act of forgiveness that empowers those who participate in this ritual.

Theory of everything (TOE): Possibility of a presently unknown fundamental theory of the universe that would incorporate quantum as well as relativity theory. Has tremendous metaphysical implications. Discussed by Ian Barbour in *Religion and Science* (San Francisco: HarperSanFrancisco, 1997), 207–9.

Tikkun: Kabbalistic notion of repair or healing. Applies to individual souls *tikkun ha'nefesh*, which is intimately related to healing the world *tikkun ha'olam*. Multiple sources, including Adin Steinsaltz, *The Thirteen Petalled Rose* (New York: Basic Books, 1980).

Two small clouds: Quote from physicist Lord Kelvin at the end of the nineteenth century that only two small issues were yet to be resolved in coming to a complete understanding of physics. These "two small clouds" led to the monumental discoveries of quantum and relativity theory. Discussed by Johnjoe McFadden in *Quantum Evolution* (New York: Norton, 2001), 139.

Notes

META-PHYSICIAN'S MOTTO

The Buddha, "*Kalama Sutra, The Instruction to the Kalamas*," trans. Soma Thera. Interpreted and discussed at: http://www.buddhistinformation.com/ida_b_wells_memorial_sutra_library/kalama_sutta.htm.

The quote is attributed to the Hindu prince Gautama Siddhartha, also known as The Buddha. It appears in *The Kalama Sutra, Sutta No. 65, Verse 15*, which tells the story of Buddha's visit to the village of Kesaputta, where he was greeted by the inhabitants, known as the Kalamas. The Kalamas ask the Buddha whose teachings they should follow. In response, he delivered a sutta that serves as an entry point to Buddhist beliefs to those unconvinced by revelatory experiences. His response, quoted in the opening of this book, has become the Buddhist charter on free thought.

Another version appears in http://en.wikipedia.org/wiki/Kalama_Sutra:

Do not go upon what has been acquired by repeated hearing; nor upon tradition; nor upon rumor; nor upon what is in a scripture; nor upon surmise; nor upon an axiom; nor upon specious reasoning; nor upon a bias towards a notion that has been pondered over; nor upon another's seeming ability; nor upon the consideration that "The monk is your teacher." (*Kalama Sutra*)

It is mentioned in many books on the Buddha, including:

Thich Nhat Hanh, *Old Path, White Clouds: Walking in the Footsteps of The Buddha* (Parallax Press, May 1999), App. III, 65.

CHAPTER 1

Lawrence LeShan, *How to Meditate* (New York: Bantam Books, 1974).

Stephen E. Braude, Ph.D., preface of *Immortal Remains* (Lanham: Rowman & Littlefield, 2003) Preface, ix–x, describing his personal experience and reaction to observing psychic phenomena.

Roger Kamenetz, *The Jew in the Lotus* (New York: HarperCollins, 1994).

William James (referring to mystical experiences: "my own constitution shuts me out from their enjoyment almost entirely, and I can only speak of them at second hand"), "Lecture XVI on Mysticism," in *The Varieties of Religious Experiences* (New York: The Modern Library, 1999).

Bertrand Russell quote: "Science Is What You Know. Philosophy Is What You Don't Know." From Alan Wood, in *Bertrand Russell: The Passionate Skeptic* (New York: Simon & Schuster, 1958).

Paul Davies, Ph.D., *The Mind of God* (New York: Touchstone, 1992), 68.

Fritjof Capra, Ph.D., *The Tao of Physics* (Boston: Shambhala, 1999).

Arnold Mindell, Ph.D., *The Quantum Mind and Healing* (Charlottesville, VA: Hampton Roads Publishing, 2004).

Einstein quotes:

Alice Calaprice, ed., *The Quotable Einstein*, 2nd rev. ed. (Princeton, NJ: Princeton University Press, 2000), quoting Einstein in a letter to a child that asked if scientists pray, January 24, 1936 (from Einstein Archive 42-601). Full quote: "Every one who is seriously involved in the pursuit of science becomes convinced that a spirit is manifest in the laws of the Universe—a spirit vastly superior to that of man, and one in the face of which we with our modest powers must feel humble."

Science, Philosophy and Religion—A Symposium (Distributed by Harper, 1941, originally published by the University of Michigan).

Scientists and belief in God sources: Edward J. Larson, *Summer for the Gods: The Scopes Trial and America's Continuing Debate over Science and Religion* (Atlanta: University of Georgia, 1997). Larson published his first findings in *Summer for the Gods*, which was awarded the 1998 Pulitzer Prize for History (also published by Harvard University Press; Reprint edition, November 15, 1998). Larson repeated the 1916 poll of scientists first conducted by James Leuba. *Research Magazine*, University of Georgia, http://www.ovpr.uga.edu/researchnews/97su/faith.html.

de Laplace quote: from *Figments of Reality: The Evolution of the Curious Mind* by Ian Stewart and Jack Cohen (Coventry, UK: University of Warwick and Cambridge, UK: Cambridge University Press, 1999).

Arnold Mindell, Ph.D., *The Quantum Mind and Healing*, 104–6.

Einstein quote: "He [God] Doesn't Play With Dice." *The New Quantum Universe*, Born, ed. Quoted from Albert Einstein in a letter to Max Born, 1926, in *The Born–Einstein Letter* (New York: Walker & Company, 1971), 159.

Quantum theory and paradoxical thinking: Richard Feynman, "The Character of Physical Law," chap. 6 in *The New Quantum Universe* (Cambridge, MA: MIT Press, 1967), 1.

Robert Roy Britt, "Dark Energy and Dark Matter—One in the Same?" Space.com, July 12, 2004.

Lawrence LeShan, *The Medium, the Mystic and the Physicist: Toward a General Theory of the Paranormal* (New York: Helios Press, 1966).

Ken Wilber, *Quantum Question: Mystical Writings of the World's Greatest Physicists* (Boston, MA: Shambhala, 1984).

CHAPTER 2

Einstein quote: Max Jammer, *Einstein and Religion* (Princeton, New Jersey: Princeton University Press, 1999), 73.

Paul Davies, *The Mind of God*.

Meditation and findings on SPECT SCAN: Andrew Newberg and Eugene D'Aquili, *Why God Won't Go Away, Brain Science and the Biology of Belief* (New York: Ballantine, 2001).

Lawrence LeShan, *The Medium, the Mystic and the Physicist.*

Ken Wilber, *Quantum Question.*

John Wheeler quote: from Nick Herbert, *Quantum Reality* (New York: Anchor Books, 1985), 29.

John von Neumann: from Herbert, *Quantum Reality*, 29.

Einstein quote: Jammer, *Einstein and Religion*, 144.

CHAPTER 3

Elisabeth Kubler-Ross, *On Life After Death* (California: Celestial Arts, 1991).

Nietzsche quote: *Nietzsche Werke: Kritische Gesamtausgabe—Also Sprach Zarathustra* (Berlin: Walter de Gruyter, June 1967). Actual quote in German: "Was nicht mich umbringt, macht mir staerker."

CHAPTER 5

Ralph Waldo Emerson quote: Edwin Doak Mead, *The Influence of Emerson* (Boston: Kessinger, 2003), 26.

Anaïs Nin quote: Quoteworld.org.

CHAPTER 6

Einstein quote: from Albert Einstein, *Ideas and Opinions* (New York: Crown, 1954) 224–227.

Dalai Lama: His Holiness the Dalai Lama, *The Universe in a Single Atom: The Convergence of Science and Spirituality* (New York: Morgan Road Books, 2005).

Wave particle duality: Tony Hey and Patrick Walters, *The New Quantum Universe* (Cambridge, UK: Cambridge University Press, 2003).

Theory of Everything (TOE): Ian Barbour, *Religion and Science* (San Francisco: HarperSanFrancisco, 1997), 207–9.

"Two small clouds" quote from physicist Lord Kelvin: Johnjoe McFadden, *Quantum Evolution* (New York: Norton, 2001), 139. At the end of the nineteenth century, only two small issues were yet to be resolved in coming to a complete understanding of physics. These "two small clouds" led to the monumental discoveries of quantum and relativity theory.

Dr. Kenneth R. Pelletier, *The Best Alternative Medicine* (New York: Fireside /Simon & Schuster, 2000).

Jane E. Brody and Denise Grady, *The New York Times Guide to Alternative Health* (New York: New York Times Books/Henry Holt, 2001).

Daniel J. Benor, M.D., *Consciousness, Bioenergy and Healing—Self-Healing and Energy Medicine for the 21st Century* (Medford, NJ: Wholistic Healing Publications, 2004).

William James, *The Varieties of Religious Experiences.*

Lawrence LeShan, *The Medium, the Mystic and the Physicist.*

Raymond Moody, *Life After Life* (New York: Bantam Books, 1975).

Kenneth Ring, *Life After Death* (New York: Coward, McCann, Geoghegan, 1980).

Peter Fenwick and Elizabeth Fenwick, *The Truth in Light* (New York: Berkley Books, 1997).

Elisabeth Kubler-Ross, *On Life After Death*.

Gary Schwartz, *The Afterlife Experiments: Breakthrough Scientific Evidence of Life After Death* (New York: Pocket Books, 2001). Psychologist Gary Schwartz has systematically studied the abilities of contemporary mediums to provide information regarding deceased loved ones. His conclusions including the use of controlled studies have been extremely favorable toward the truth of the mediums' experiences.

CHAPTER 7

Sir Arthur Eddington quote: from the quotation page of www.quotationpage.com.

Theodore Roethke, "The Waking," in *The Collected Poems of Theodore Roethke* (New York: Doubleday, 1953), 49.

David Deutch, "Quantum Theory and the Observation of Phenomena," *The Fabric of Reality* (New York: Penguin, 1997), 76, 69, 147, 224.

CHAPTER 8

Einstein quote: Attributed to *NY Times Magazine*, November 9, 1930, as wikiquotes.com.

Robert Todd Carroll, *The Skeptic's Dictionary* (New York: John Wiley & Sons, Inc., 2003), 306, explanation of *Pseudoscience*.

John Horgan, *The End of Science* (New York: Broadway Books, 1996), 5–6.

Johnjoe McFadden, *Quantum Evolution*, 99–101. Refers to the anthropic principle—the concept that the existence of the physical universe as we know it is incredibly unlikely based on the laws of probability and the magnitude of multiple physical constants.

CHAPTER 9

Ralph Waldo Emerson, *Natural History of Intellect and Other Papers: With a General Index to Emerson's Collected Works* (Boston, Adamant Media, 2001), 17.

William James quote: from Helen Granat, *Wisdom through the Ages: A Collection of Favorite Quotations*, 1st ed. (Victoria, BC, Canada: Miklen Press, 1998), 19.

David Chalmers, *The Conscious Mind: In Search of a Fundamental Theory* (Oxford: Oxford University Press, 1996).

CHAPTER 10

Mae West Quote: John A. Simpson, *The Concise Oxford Dictionary of Proverbs* (Oxford: Oxford University Press, 1992), 258.

Matthieu Ricard, *Happiness: A Guide to Developing Life's Most Important Skill*, trans. Jesse Browner (New York: Little, Brown, 2003).

Jonathan Haidt, *The Happiness Hypothesis: Finding Modern Truth in Ancient Wisdom* (New York: Basic Books, 2006).

CHAPTER 11

Paul Davies, *The Mind of God*, 231–32.

Theodore Roethke, "In a Dark Time," in Davies, *The Mind of God*, 231.

CHAPTER 12

Lawrence LeShan, *The Medium, the Mystic and the Physicist*, ix.

S. E. Hodes quote: This is a quote by the author.

William James, M. (Boston, MA: Adamant Media, 2001) 17.D., *The Varieties of Religious Experiences*.

Raymond Moody, *Life After Life*.

Matthew Alper, *The God Part of the Brain* (Brooklyn, NY: Rogue, 2001). Alper offers convincing arguments that mankind seems to be genetically predisposed to religious belief. He refers to the work of Andrew Newberg and Eugene D'Aquili at the Nuclear Medicine division at the University of Pennsylvania who used SPECT (single positron emission computed tomography) to demonstrate that spiritual/mystical experiences are located within physical areas and structures of the brain. William James, M.D., *The Varieties of Religious Experiences*. Considered the Father of American psychology, he wrote about spirituality and paranormal experiences, and said that to the actual individual who has had a deeply personal, highly subjective experience, there is no doubt it is real.

CHAPTER 13

Voltaire quote: from Richard Webster, *Practical Guide to Past-Life Memories* (St. Paul, MN: Llewellyn, 2001), 107.

Bhagavad-Gita quote: A. C. Prabhupada, *Bhagavad-Gita As It Is* (Alachua, FL: Bhaktivedanta Book Trust, vinyl cover edition, 1989), 95.

Information on the Wiccan faith: Excerpt on Wicca from *Religious Requirements and Practices of Certain Selected Groups: A Handbook for Chaplains* (The U.S. Department of the Army, first published in 1978; published in 2001 under the same name). Source: www.religioustolerance.org/wic_usbk.htm.

Ian Stevenson, M.D., *Children Who Remember* (Virgina: The University Press of Virginia, 1987).

Ian Stevenson, M.D., *Where Reincarnation and Biology Intersect* (Westport, CT: Praeger, 1997). He has been documenting case studies from children who remember past lives in extraordinary ways and he has produced compelling evidence in his studies.

Brian Weiss, M.D., *Many Lives, Many Masters* (New York: Fireside, 1988).

Michael Newton, *Journey of Souls* (St. Paul, MN: Llewellyn, 1994), 399.

Michael Newton, *Destiny of Souls* (St. Paul, MN: Llewellyn, 2000).

Michael Newton, *Life Between Lives* (St. Paul, MN: Llewellyn, 2004).

CHAPTER 14

Fyodor Dostoevsky, *A Writer's Diary: 1873–1876* (Northwestern University Press, reprint ed., 1997).

Joseph Campbell, *The Power of Myth* (New York: Broadway Books, reissue ed., 1988), 151–52.

Fusae Kanda, writing in an entry titled "Behind the Sensationalism: Images of a Decaying Corpse in Japanese Buddhist Art" from *The Art Bulletin* and published on FindArticles.com March 2005, says, "the practice of contemplating on a decaying corpse was adopted widely by monks regardless of their sectarian affiliations" and that it was "frequently mentioned in Buddhist sutras." http://findarticles.com/p/articles/mi_m0422/is_1_87/ai_n13592441/pg_2.

CHAPTER 15

The Buddha quote: Houston Smith, *The World's Religions: Our Great Wisdom Traditions* (San Francisco: HarperSanFrancisco, 1991), 98.

CHAPTER 16

Mahatma Gandhi quote: R. K. Prabhu & U. R. Rao, eds., *The Mind of Mahatma Gandhi* (Ahmedabad, India: Jitendra T. Desai, 4th reprint, 1996).

CHAPTER 17

The Lord's Prayer, found in Gospel of Matthew 6:9–13 and Luke 11:2–4.
Passover Seder: Scherkan Zlotowitz, in and Nosson Scherman and Avie Gold, eds., *Family Haggadah: Hagadah Shel Pesah* (Brooklyn, NY: Artscroll Mesorah Series, 1981).

CHAPTER 18

Wayne Dyer quote, *Real Magic: Creating Miracles in Everyday Life* (New York: Harper Paperbacks, 2001), 92.

CHAPTER 19

Estelle Frankel, *Sacred Therapy: Jewish Spiritual Teachings on Emotional Healing and Inner Wholeness* (Boston: Shambhala, 2005), 4.
Ram Dass, *Still Here: Embracing Aging, Changing, Dying* (New York: Riverhead Books, 2000), 5.

CHAPTER 20

Rabbi Joseph Gelberman quote: Spoken at the New Synagogue in New York City on the occasion of his 95th birthday, May 4, 2007.
Viktor Frankl, *Man's Search for Meaning* (New York: Washington Square Press, 1985).

CHAPTER 21

Dalai Lama quote: from Susan Santucci, in *Converging Paths: Lessons of Compassion, Tolerance and Understanding from East and West* (Boston: Turtle, 2003), 91.
Dalai Lama quote: Dalai Lama and Howard C. Cutler, *The Art of Happiness: A Handbook for Living* (New York: Riverhead Books, 1998), 3.

CHAPTER 22

Scriptural Quote: Psalm 34:18, New International Version of the Bible.

CHAPTER 23

Carl Jung, *Memories, Dreams and Reflections* (New York: Vintage, 1989).

CHAPTER 24

Sir William Osler quote: W. Grant Thomas quotes "the Father of Modern Medicine," Osler, in *The Placebo Effect and Health* (Amherst, NY: Prometheus Books, 2005), 23.

CHAPTER 25

Dennis Waitley quote: from Steve Ryals, *Drunk with Wonder: Awakening to the God Within* (Ukiah, CA: Rock Creek Press), 87.

Obesity and health risk: Statistics available in "Common Risk Factors: Overweight and Obesity" prepared by the New York State Department for the Aging. http://agingwell. state.ny.us/prevention/overweight.htm

Jewish Beauty Prayer: Hayim Halevy Donin, *To Be a Jew: A Guide to Jewish Observance in Contemporary Life* (Basic Books, 2001), 170.

CHAPTER 26

Rabbi Menachem Schneerson quote: Compiled by Tzvi Freeman, *Bringing Heaven Down to Earth: Meditations and Everyday Wisdom from the Teachings of the Rebbe, Menachem Schneerson* (Holbrook, MA: Adams Media, 1996), 13.

Einstein quote: from Barbara De Angelis, in *How Did I Get Here?: Finding Your Way to Renewed Hope and Happiness When Life and Love Take* (New York: St. Martin's Press, 2005), 277.

CHAPTER 27

Søren Kierkegaard quote: *Soren Kierkegaard's Journals and Papers, Part 1 (Autobiographical) Part One (1829–1848)* (Indiana University Press, August 1978)

Teilhard de Chardin quote: "We are not human beings having a spiritual experience, but rather spiritual beings having a human experience." Widely used anonomously and originally attributed to him; source unknown.

Ram Dass quote: Ram Dass, from Barbara DeAngelis, *In Touch Magazine.*

Viktor Frankl, from *Man's Search for Meaning.*

Rabbi Joseph Gelberman, founder of the New Synagogue in New York City, often shares at his monthly service that he lost his wife and young child in the Holocaust, yet has based his life on the premise that we are meant to be joyous, excited about life, and loving—despite what hardships may come. He often quotes from Psalm 23 ("Yea, though I walk through the valley of the shadow of death, I will fear no evil") and talks about how continuing the journey despite life's difficulties is the point. Giving up is not an option.

Rabbi Harold Kushner, *The Lord Is My Shepherd* (New York: Knopf, 2003). He commented on the next phrase of Psalm 23 that states, "for Thou art with me." He noted that God does not promise that life is fair or easy, only that we would not have to face it alone.

Bibliography

Alper, Michael. *The God Part of the Brain*. Brooklyn, NY: Rogue Press, 2001.

Anderson, George and Andrew Barone. *Lessons from the Light*. New York: Berkley Books, 1999.

Archangel, Diane. *Afterlife Encounters*. Charlottesville, VA: Hampton Roads, 2005.

Atwater, P.M.H. *We Live Forever*. Virginia Beach: A.R.E. Press, 2004.

Audi, Robert, Ed. *The Cambridge Dictionary of Philosophy*. Cambridge: Cambridge University Press, 2001.

Barbour, Ian G. *Religion and Science*. San Francisco: HarperSanFrancisco, 1997.

Barrett, William. *Death of the Soul*. Garden City, NY: Anchor Press, 1986.

Batie, Howard. *Healing Body, Mind and Spirit*. St. Paul, MN: Llewellyn, 2004.

Becker, Earnest. *The Denial of Death*. New York: Free Press Paperbacks, 1973.

Benor, Daniel J. *Spiritual Healing, A Scientific Validation of a Healing Revolution*. Southfield, MI: Vision, 2001.

———. *Consciousness, Bioenergy and Healing*. Medford, NJ: Wholistic Healing, 2004.

Blum, Deborah. *Ghosthunters*. New York: The Penguin Press, 2006.

Borysenko, Joan and Miroslave Borysenko. *The Power of the Mind to Heal*. Carlsbad, CA: Hay House, 1994.

Braude, Stephen. *Immortal Remains*. Lanham, MD: Rowman & Littlefield, 2003.

Britt, Robert Roy. *Dark Energy and Dark Matter—One in the Same?* Space.com, July 12, 2004.

Brody, Jane and Denise Grady. *The New York Times Guide to Alternative Health*. New York: The New Times Books, Holt, 2001.

Capra, Fritjof. *The Tao of Physics*. Boston, MA: Shambhala, 1991.

———. *The Web of Life*. New York: Doubleday, 1996.

Cerminara, Gina. *Many Mansions: The Edgar Cayce Story on Reincarnation*. New York: Signet, 1999.

Collins, Francis. *The Language of God: A Scientist Presents Evidence for Belief*. New York: Free Press, 2006.

Cooper, David. *God Is a Verb*. New York: Riverhead Books, 1997.

———. *A Heart of Stillness*. Woodstock, VT: Skylight Paths, 1999.

Currie, Ian. *Visions of Immortality*. Shaftesbury, Dorset: Element Books, 1998.

Dass, Ram. *Be Here Now*. New York: Crown, 1971.

———. *Still Here*. New York: Riverhead Books, 2000.

Davies, Paul. *God and the New Physics*. New York: Touchstone, 1983.

Davies, Paul and John Gribben. *The Matter Myth*. New York: Touchstone, 1992.

Dawkins, Richard. *Unweaving the Rainbow*. Boston, MA: Mariner Books, 1998.

———. *The God Delusion*. New York: Houghton Mifflin, 2006

Dossey, Larry. *Recovering the Soul*. New York: Bantam Books, 1989.

———. *Reinventing Medicine*. San Francisco: HarperSanFrancisco, 1999.

Ducasse, C.J. *A Critical Examination of the Belief in Life after Death*. Spingfield, IL: Thomas, 1961.

Dyer, Wayne W. *Wisdom of the Ages*. New York: HarperCollins Publishers, 1998.

Easterbrook, Greg. "The New Convergence." Article in *Wired* 10.12, December 2002.

Edward, John. *One Last Time*. New York: Berkley Books, 1998.

Einstein, Albert. *Ideas and Opinions*. New York: Three Rivers Press, 1982.

Epstein, Mark. *Going to Pieces without Falling Apart*. New York: Broadway Books, 1999.

Fenwick, Peter and Elizabeth Fenwick. *The Truth in Light*. New York: Berkley Books, 1997.

Fitzgerald, Astrid. *Being, Consciousness, Bliss*. Great Barrington, MA: Lindisfarne Books, 2001.

Fontana, David. *Is There an Afterlife?* Dershot Lodge, Park Lane, UK: O Books, 2005.

Frankel, Estelle. *Sacred Therapy*. Boston, MA: Shambhala, 2005.

Frankel, Tamar. *The Gift of Kabbalah*. Woodstock, VT: Jewish Lights, 2004.

Frankl, Viktor. *Man's Search for Meaning*. New York: Washington Square Press, 1985.

Friedman, Norman. *The Hidden Domain*. Eugene, OR: The Woodbridge Group, 1997.

Gallagher, Winifred. *Spiritual Genius*. New York: Random House, 2001.

Gerber, Richard. *Vibrational Medicine*. Rochester, VT: Bear & Co, 2001.

Gershom, Rabbi Yonassan. *Beyond the Ashes*. Virginia Beach, VA: A.R.E. Press, 1992.

Goldberg, Bruce. *Peaceful Transition*. St. Paul, MN: Llewellyn, 1997.

Goodenough, Ursula. *The Sacred Depths of Nature*. Oxford University Press, 1998.

Gordon, Richard. *Quantum Touch*. Berkeley, CA: North Atlantic Books, 2002.

Goswami, Amit. *The Self Aware Universe*. New York: Penguin Putnam, 1993.

Greene, Brian. *The Elegant Universe*. New York: W.W. Norton, 1999.

Greenspan, Miriam. *Healing through the Dark Emotions, the Wisdom of Grief, Fear, and Despair*. Boston, MA: Shambhala, 2004.

Haidt, Jonathan. *The Happiness Hypothesis*. New York: Basic Books, 2006.

Heschel, Abraham Joshua. *I Asked for Wonder*. Ed. Samuel H. Dresner. New York: Crossroad, 1997.

Holland, John. *Born Knowing*. Carlsbad, CA: Hay House, 2003.

Holzer, Hans. *Life Beyond*. Chicago, IL: Contemporary Books, 1994.

———. *The Supernatural*. Franklin Lakes, NJ: New Page Books, 2003.

James, William. *The Varieties of Religious Experience*. New York: The Modern Library, 1999.

Kafatos, Menas and Robert Nadeau. *The Conscious Universe*. New York: Springer, 1990.

Kamentz, Roger. *The Jew in the Lotus*. San Francisco: HarperSanFrancisco, 1994.

———. *Stalking Elijah*. San Francisco: HarperSanFrancisco, 1997.

Kaplan, Aryeh. *Meditation and Kabbalah*. York Beach, Maine: Samuel Weiser, 1982.

Kubler-Ross, Elisabeth. *On Life after Death*. Berkley, CA: Celestial Arts, 1991.

Kurtz, Paul, Ed. *Science and Religion*. Amherst, NY: Prometheus Books, 2003.

Kushner, Harold S. *The Lord Is My Shepherd*. New York: Alfred A. Knopf, 2003.

Lama, Dalai. *Essential Teachings*. London: Souvenir Press, 1999.

———. *The Universe in a Single Atom*. New York: Morgan Road Books, 2005.

LeShan, Lawrence. *How to Meditate*. New York: Bantam Books, 1974.

———. *The Medium, the Mystic and the Physicist.* New York: Helios Press, 2003.

Malin, Shimon. *Nature Loves to Hide.* New York: Oxford University Press, 2001.

Margulies, Lynn and Dorion Sagan. *What Is Life?* Berkeley, CA: University of California Press, 1995.

Matheson, Richard. *What Dreams May Come?* New York: Tom Doherty Associates, 1978.

Matt, Daniel. *The Essential Kabbalah.* Edison, NJ: Castle Books, 1995.

———. *God and the Big Bang.* Woodstock, VT: Jewish Lights Books, 1996.

McGraw, John J. *Brain and Belief: An Exploration of the Human Soul.* Del Mar, CA: Aegis Press, 2004.

McMoneagle, Joseph. *Mind Trek.* Charlottesville, VA: Hampton Roads, 1997.

McTaggart, Lynne. *The Field, the Quest for the Secret Force of the Universe.* New York: HarperCollins, 2002.

Midgely, Mary. *Science and Poetry.* London: Routledge, 2001.

Miller, Sukie. *After Death.* New York: Simon & Schuster, 1997.

Mindell, Arthur. *Quantum Mind.* Oregon: Lao Tse Press, 2000.

Moody, Raymond. *Life after Life.* New York: Bantam Books, 1975.

———. *Reunions.* New York: Ivy Books, 1993.

———. *The Last Laugh.* Charlottesville, VA: Hampton Roads, 1999.

Moody, Raymond and Diane Archangel. *Life after Loss.* San Francisco: HarperSanFrancisco, 2001.

Morris, Thomas V., Ed. *God and the Philosophers.* New York: Oxford University Press, 1994.

Myss, Caroline. *Anatomy of the Spirit.* New York: Three Rivers Press, 1996.

Nesse, Randolf and George Williams. *Why We Get Sick.* Vintage Books, 1996.

Newberg, Andrew and Eugene D'Aquili. *The Mystical Mind.* Minnesota: Fortress Press, 1999.

———. *Why God Won't Go Away, Brain Science and the Biology of Belief.* New York: Ballantine Books, 2001.

Newton, Michael. *Journey of Souls.* St. Paul, MN: Llewellyn, 1994.

———. *Destiny of Souls.* St. Paul, MN: Llewellyn, 2000.

———. *Life between Lives.* St. Paul, MN: Llewellyn, 2004.

Osis, Karlis and Erlendur Haradlsson. *At the Hour of Death.* Norwalk, CT: Hastings House, third edition, 1997.

Pearsall, Paul. *The Hearts Code.* New York: Broadway Books, 1998.

Pelletier, Kenneth R. *The Best Alternative Medicine.* New York: Simon & Schuster, 2001.

Pert, Candace. *Molecules of Emotion.* New York: Scribner, 1997.

Pollan, Michael. *The Botany of Desire.* New York: Random House, 2001.

Powell, Corey S. *God in the Equation.* London: Free Press, 2002.

Radin, Dean. *The Conscious Universe.* San Francisco: HarperEdge, 1997

Ramachandran, V.S. *A Brief Tour of Human Consciousness.* New York: Pi Press, 2004.

Ramo, Chet. *Skeptics and True Believers.* New York: MJF Books, 1998.

Raphael, Simcha Paull. *Jewish Views on the Afterlife.* Northvale, NJ: Jason Aronson, 1996.

Ricard, Matthieu. *Happiness: A Guide to Developing Life's Most Important Skill,* trans. Jesse Browner. New York: Little, Brown and Company, 2003.

Ricard, Mattheiu and Trinh Xuan Thuan. *The Quantum and the Lotus.* New York: Crown Publishers, 2001.

Ring, Kenneth. *Life after Death.* New York: Coward, McCann, Geoghegan, 1980.

Rinpoche, Chockyi Nyima. *Medicine and Compassion.* Boston: Wisdom, 2004.

Rinpoche, Sogyal. *The Tibetan Book of Living and Dying.* New York: HarperCollins, 1992.

Roomer, Barbara. *Blessing in Disguise.* St. Paul, MN: Llewellyn, 2000.

Russell, Peter. *The Science of God.* Novato, CA: New World Library, 2002.

Sabom, Michael. *Light and Death.* Grand Rapids, MI: Zondervan, 1998.

Salzberg, Sharon. *Loving Kindness.* Boston, MA: Shambhala Classics, 2002.

Schneerson, Menachem. *Bringing Heaven Down to Earth.* Holbrook, MA: Adams Media Corporation, 1999.

Schroder, Gerald. *The Science of God.* New York: Broadway Books, 1997.

Schwartz, Gary. *The Afterlife Experiments.* New York: Pocket Books, 2002.

Shanor, Karen Nesbitt. *The Emerging Mind.* Los Angeles: Renaissance Books, 1999.

Shulman, Jason. *Kabbalistic Healing.* Rochester, VT: Inner Traditions, 2004.

Solomon, Philip and Hans Holzer. *Beyond Death.* Charlottesville, VA: Hampton Roads, 2001.

Solomon, Robert. *Spirituality for the Skeptic.* New York: Oxford University Press, 2002.

Spitz, Elie Kaplan. *Does the Soul Survive.* Woodstock, VT: Jewish Lights, 2000.

Steinsaltz, Adin. *The Thirteen Petalled Rose.* New York: Basic Books, 1980.

Stevenson, Ian. *Children Who Remember.* Charlottesville, VA: The University Press of Virginia, 1987.

————. *Where Reincarnation and Biology Intersect.* Westport, CT: Praeger, 1997.

Stewart, Ian and Jack Cohen. *Figments of Reality.* Cambridge: Cambridge University Press, 1997

Strobel, Lee. *The Case for a Creator.* Grand Rapids, MI: Zondervan, 2004.

Sylvia, Claire. *A Change of Heart.* New York: Warner Books, 1997.

Talbot, Michael. *The Holographic Universe.* New York: HarperPerrenial, 1991.

Teasdale, Wayne. *The Mystic Heart.* Novato, CA: New World Library, 2001.

Thomas, Lewis. *The Lives of a Cell.* New York: The Viking Press, 1974.

Thurman, Robert. *Infinite Life.* New York: Riverhead Books, 2004.

Tipler, Frank. *The Physics of Immortality.* New York: Anchor Books, 1994.

Weiss, Brian. *Many Lives, Many Masters.* New York: Fireside, 1988.

Whitehead, Alfred North. *Adventures of Ideas.* New York: The Free Press, 1967.

Wilbur, Ken. *The Essential Ken Wilber.* Boston, MA: Shambhala, 1998.

————. *The Eye of the Spirit.* Boston, MA: Shambhala, 1998.

————. *Quantum Questions.* Boston, MA: Shambhala, 2001.

————. *Integral Spirituality.* Boston: Integral Books, 2006.

Wilson, Colin. *After Life.* St.Paul, MN: Llewellyn, 2000.

Zammit, Victor. *A Lawyer Presents the Case for the Afterlife.* E-book online at www.victorzammit.com.

Zukav, Gary. *The Dancing Wu Li Maters.* New York: Bantam Books, 1979.

Index

About the Author

STEVEN E. HODES, M.D., is a board-certified gastroenterologist with over twenty-five years' private practice based in Edison and Old Bridge, New Jersey. He received his medical degree from the Albert Einstein College of Medicine, and did his gastroenterology fellowship at Mount Sinai Hospital in New York. He also has a degree in religious studies from Franklin and Marshall College.

In addition to his medical practice, he has devoted himself to speaking and writing about metaphysics and healing, with an eye toward helping people regain their health, strength, and the ability to explore life's challenges from a more spiritual perspective.

Dr. Hodes is a teacher of metaphysics and lecturer on many compelling spiritual topics. He's been instructor of "Contemporary Metaphysics and Healing" at Brookdale Community College in Lincroft, New Jersey, since 2002. He also lectures for the 92nd Street Y in New York on "Science and Spirituality."

His articles have been published in dozens of healing-oriented magazines such as *Townsend Letter for Doctors and Patients*, *International Journal of Healing and Caring*, *Well Being Journal*, *Alternatives Magazine*, *Whole Living Journal*, *In Light Times*, *Of Spirit*, *Spirit Crossing*, *Soulful Living*, *Pathways Within*, *Inspiration Line*, *Sure Woman* and many others. Visit his blog "Physician to Meta-Physician" at www.meta-md.com.